Also by Shaun Assael

Sex, Lies, and Headlocks: The Real Story of Vince McMahon and World Wrestling Entertainment (with Mike Mooneyham)

Wide Open: Days and Nights on the NASCAR Tour

STEROID

NATION

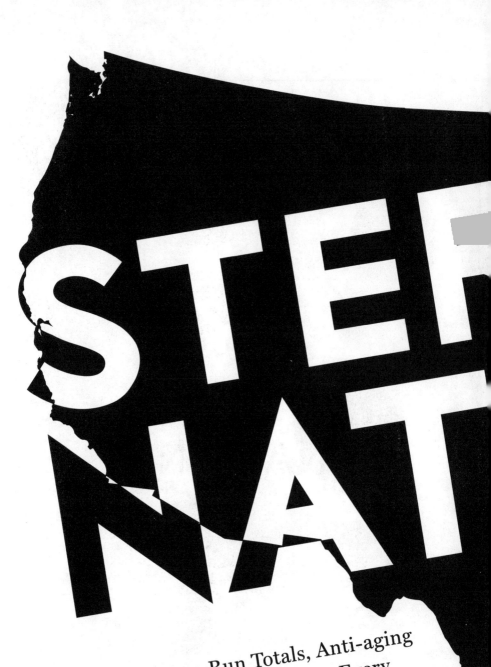

STER
NAT

 Juiced Home Run Totals, Anti-aging
Miracles, and a Hercules in Every
High School: The Secret History of
America's True Drug Addiction

Shaun Assael

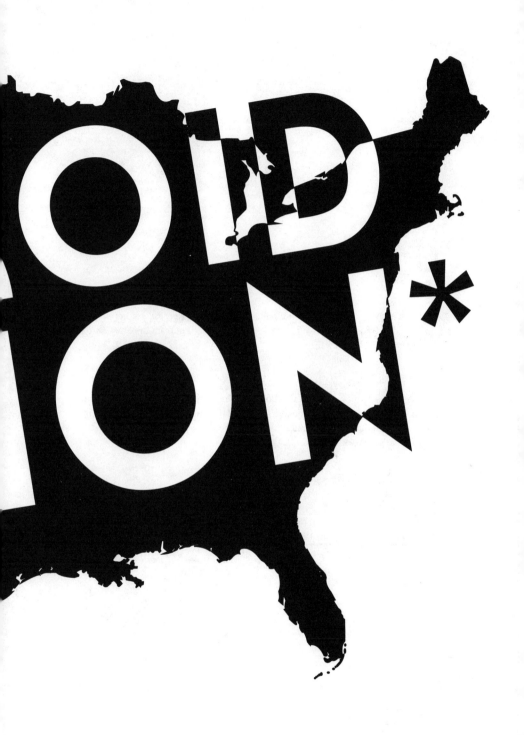

To Ellen and Jake, the biggest believers

"One cannot violate the promptings of one's nature without having that nature recoil upon itself."

JACK LONDON
White Fang

—

"And still the figure had no face by which he might know it; even in his dreams, it had no face, or one that baffled him and melted before his eyes; and thus it was that there sprang up and grew apace in [his] mind a singularly strong, an almost inordinate, curiosity to behold the features of the real Mr. Hyde."

ROBERT LOUIS STEVENSON
The Strange Case of Dr. Jekyll and Mr. Hyde

CONTENTS

PART I

PART II

PART III

THE STEROID NATION

THE GURUS

DAN DUCHAINE: Author of the *Underground Steroid Handbook*. Served two federal prison sentences for drug dealing while becoming known internationally as The Guru.

MICHAEL ZUMPANO: Co-author of the *Underground Steroid Handbook*. Broke with Duchaine in 1983 to open a vitamin and supplement company. Later sponsored Mark McGwire.

BILL PHILLIPS: Former bodybuilder. Founded *Muscle Media* magazine in 1992 and hired Duchaine to write a column about steroids. Built the supplement company EAS into a giant, based on the popularity of creatine. Sold EAS for huge profit and went on to write best-selling self-help books.

VICTOR CONTE: Ex-musician who turned a small San Francisco blood-testing lab, BALCO, into a notorious pipeline for designer steroids from 2000-2003. Served four months in federal prison.

PATRICK ARNOLD: Chemist and supplement company owner whose secret production of designer steroids earned him a three-month prison sentence in the BALCO case in 2006.

ARNOLD SCHWARZENEGGER: Film actor and spiritual leader of bodybuilding's Arnoldistas. Now Governor of California.

THE UNDERGROUND

TONY FITTON: Described as "perhaps the largest steroid dealer in the world" when he was arrested in 1984.

DAVID JENKINS: At 19, won an Olympic silver medal in the 4x100-meter relay in 1972; convicted of conspiracy and related steroids charges in 1988 with Duchaine and sentenced to seven years. Went on to open a successful supplement company.

WILLIAM DILLON: Former Mr. Collegiate Illinois bodybuilding champion and Gold's Gym regular. Joined Jenkins and Duchaine in the Mexican smuggling operation.

JUAN MACKLIS: Mexican factory owner who counterfeited steroids for the Duchaine group. Still under indictment in the U.S., he is considered a fugitive.

ALBERTO SALTIEL-COHEN: Mexican veterinary steroid manufacturer, arrested in San Diego in 2005 as part of a Drug Enforcement Administration crackdown on smuggling. Stood accused of producing 70 percent of the veterinary steroids smuggled into the United States from Mexico for human use.

THE SALESMEN

ANTHONY ALMADA: Biochemist who started EAS with a partner in 1992 after discovering the muscle-building properties of creatine. Merged with Bill Phillips in 1994, and sold his lucrative stake in the company to Phillips two years later.

LARRY WOOD: Life extension and anti-aging disciple. Convicted with Dan Duchaine of distributing GHB in 1992.

STAN ANTOSH: San Francisco personal trainer who helped invent and market Andro. Sentenced to three years in federal prison on charges related to his earlier manufacturing of GHB.

BRUCE KNELLER: Former Massachusetts nurse who became Dan Duchaine's research assistant and later an influential designer of steroidal supplements. Began serving a two-year prison term in 2007 after pleading guilty to charges of steroid possession and distribution.

THE WATCHDOGS

DON CATLIN: Director, UCLA Olympic Analysis Lab, 1983-2007. America's leading steroid hunter.

ALEXANDRE DE MÉRODE: Belgian prince (now deceased) and longtime chairman of the International Olympic Committee's medical commission.

TERRY MADDEN: Founding CEO of the United States Anti-Doping Agency (USADA), 2000-2007.

LORI LEWIS: Crusading mother who single-handedly uncovered steroid use at her son's Texas high school. Helped bring mandatory high school steroid testing to Texas.

DON HOOTON: Marketing executive turned anti-steroid activist after his son Taylor committed suicide in 2003. Hooton blamed steroids for the 17-year-old pitcher's death.

DICK POUND: Chairman, World Anti-Doping Agency (WADA).

DENNIS DEGAN: National Steroid Investigation Coordinator, Food and Drug Administration, 1983-1993.

PHILLIP HALPERN: Assistant U.S. Attorney, San Diego.

DAVID KESSLER: Commissioner, Food and Drug Administration 1990-1997.

JEFF NOVITZKY: Special agent, Internal Revenue Service. Starting with the BALCO case, spearheaded multiple probes of performance-enhancing drugs in sports.

JACK MACGREGOR: Special Agent, Drug Enforcement Administration. Targeted Mexican steroid manufacturers with undercover case, Operation Gear Grinder.

THE GADFLIES

CHARLIE FRANCIS: Ex-coach for Ben Johnson whose admitted steroid peddling electrified the Dubin Commission when he testified in 1989.

HOWARD JACOBS: Ex-triathlete turned defense lawyer, who handled every important doping case to emerge from the U.S. Anti-Doping Agency, including those of Tim Montgomery and Floyd Landis.

LOREN ISRAELSEN: Salt Lake City attorney and supplement industry lobbyist. After helping win the passage of DSHEA, backed a 2004 bill that banned Andro and its successors.

THE POLITICIANS

SENATOR ORRIN HATCH: Utah Republican who was a key sponsor of the Dietary Supplement Health and Education Act of 1994 (DSHEA).

SENATOR JOSEPH BIDEN: Delaware Democrat who sponsored the landmark 1990 bill that made steroids a controlled substance and the 2004 law that banned steroidal supplements such as Andro.

REPRESENTATIVE HENRY WAXMAN: Southern California Democrat who fought against DSHEA and spearheaded hearings on steroids in baseball.

THE STARS

BEN JOHNSON: Stripped of the 1988 Olympic 100-meter gold medal in track after drug tests showed presence of stanozonol. Claimed he was the victim of a setup.

LYLE ALZADO: Played for the Denver Broncos, Cleveland Browns, and Los Angeles Raiders from 1971-1985. Attempted a comeback in 1990. Died of cancer in 1992. Blamed steroid use for his death.

MARK MCGWIRE: Played with the Oakland A's and St. Louis Cardinals from 1986-2001. Broke Roger Maris's single-season home run record with 70 in 1998. Later refused to talk about steroid use in baseball during hearings before Congress.

JOSE CANSECO: Former American League MVP and teammate of Mark McGwire. Implicated McGwire as a steroid user in his book, *Juiced*.

BILL ROMANOWSKI: Star of the Denver Broncos and EAS pitchman, who used his appearance in Super Bowl XXXII to gain notoriety for Bill Phillips. While playing for the Raiders in 2003, tested positive for the designer steroid THG.

TIM MONTGOMERY: Became the fastest man in the world in 2002 with a 9.78 time in the 100-meter race. The record was later expunged, and a two-year ban issued, after documents seized in the BALCO raid showed he took designer steroids.

BARRY BONDS: Seven-time National League MVP. The single-season home run leader and career home run leader. Implicated as a steroid user during the BALCO case although he has denied ever taking them.

FLOYD LANDIS: American cyclist accused of doping after a dramatic come-from-behind win in the 2006 Tour de France.

INTRODUCTION

Dan Duchaine rode his scooter past the roller girls, the Valley kids, and the wannabe rockers on the Venice Beach boardwalk, until he finally arrived at the Mecca of American bodybuilding, Gold's Gym. Parking his bike, he listened to the sound of weight machines coming from inside. They clanged in an inchoate rhythm, creating a drumbeat that was, like jazz, at once chaotic and determined. In the five years since Gold's was made famous by Arnold Schwarzenegger in *Pumping Iron*, it had become a mix of high and low culture: part tourist destination, part celebrity hot spot, part dumbbell speakeasy. People came to Gold's to reinvent themselves, and in that regard Dan Duchaine was no different from anyone else.

He had been on his own since he was 13, or, if you looked at it another way, forever. Taken in by a pair of Maine mill workers who couldn't have a child of their own, he watched his adoptive mother drop dead shortly after his 10th birthday, and his dad two years later. Abandoned for a second time, he raised himself in their modest bungalow cottage, visited occasionally by his aunt and the grandparents who lived a block away and who couldn't figure out how they had been saddled with a child who acted unlike anyone else in the town of Westbrook. He pushed the limits of his school's dress code with Nehru jackets and berets, and as soon as he got a driver's license, he tooled around in a 1959 Impala that his father had left in the garage. Among the people in Westbrook, it was generally agreed that Dan Duchaine was the most flamboyant.

Still, it was hard to top the crowd that filled Gold's this Sunday morning. In one corner, Duchaine spied the muscle-bound twins with mullets who called themselves the Barbarian Brothers. In another, he saw Lisa Lyon, a bodybuilding diva who arrived for her workout in the skintight leather dress and spiked collar that she had worn the night before. This was the in-crowd, the Arnoldistas. And looking at them, Duchaine felt acutely aware of his own station as a wannabe. After four years studying drama at Boston University, and a few more spinning his wheels at a bike shop in Maine, he wasn't going to be the famous actor the locals in Westbrook had expected. But that didn't mean that he still couldn't look for a stage.

Drugs like Deca-Durabolin and Dianabol had changed Duchaine. He had started taking them in college in the mid-1970s and watched the gawky kid from Maine disappear. At 29, he still wasn't good looking. His face was too awkward for that. His eyes were set a bit too closely to the bridge of his nose, one slightly higher than the other. His lips were thin and pursed, his ears low-hanging orbs. Even his black hair, which fell over his head like a helmet, defied styling. Yet he had found a life posing in small-time bodybuilding contests around Boston that finally allowed him to put his acting skills to use. His body, never the most chiseled, somehow became graceful, his look searching and intense.

But he had taken things as far as he could on his own, and now had come to the one place where he could take them further. A small group was gathered in the middle of the gym, and he wove his way past the weight machines to join them. They were gathered for a class that the Muscle Beach cognoscenti affectionately called Sunday School, where once a week anyone could drop in and tune up.

The man who was teaching the class was everything Duchaine was not. Mike Zumpano was a strapping, good-looking 23-year-old with flowing black hair and an easy manner that belied an eagle eye for the scene. Zumpano knew that bodybuilding competitions paid nothing compared to what someone could make on the side at Gold's, which was why a workout was never just a workout. Sometimes, it served as an advertisement for the drugs that fueled it, sometimes as a come-on for sex. More than a few bodybuilders supported themselves by letting rich studio executives perform favors on them in the backs of limousines with tinted windows or allowing "schmoes" to massage them for a few hundred bucks.

From his spot at the reception desk, Zumpano was their musclehead maître d'hôtel. One day, he picked up the gym's phone to hear a woman go on about how her ex-husband was ruining her life. Was there anyone, she asked, who could rough him up for just $200? Zumpano yelled, "I got a hardship case here. Anyone interested?" A 400-pound regular took the gig.

Gold's had plenty of other secrets. Zumpano knew pharmaceutical reps from the major drug companies who stopped by periodically to make side money selling drug samples to the lifters. And he knew those lifters' secrets. There was the woman who begged him to let her in past midnight so she could work out in the nude. (It happened when she was strung out on heroin.) And there was the friendly cocaine dealer who gave free samples to a third of the bodybuilders, eagerly getting them hooked; when they couldn't afford to buy any more, he traded them drugs for information about where their sugar daddies kept their expensive cars. Then he sold the information to a mob-run theft ring.

Keeping a protective eye over things, Zumpano zeroed in on Duchaine as he sat on the edge of a weight bench. He had seen the newcomer around the gym a few times before; typical easterner, fast-talking and fidgety, he thought. Then he passed around a flyer and watched Duchaine eagerly grab for it. As Zumpano talked about the sources of information about steroids that he had listed on the sheet, he watched Duchaine write notes at a feverish pace. When the class ended, Duchaine walked up to him.

"How about I buy you breakfast?" he asked. Zumpano, who was a little hungry, agreed.

As they dug into steaming plates of eggs at Rose Café, Zumpano could see that Duchaine was every bit the operator that he had imagined. Some people reveal themselves slowly. Duchaine was in a race to say as much about himself as he could. He was living on the outskirts of town with his wife, Lee, who had followed him from Maine. For now, he was working as a process server "until I can get unemployment." And although Duchaine did most of the prattling, Zumpano had the distinct feeling that he was being measured for something. But what?

It soon became clearer as the weeks passed. As Duchaine became a regular at Sunday School, Zumpano began to look forward to their breakfasts. Duchaine was odd but endearingly so. For one thing, he loved turn-of-the-century recumbent bicycles and frequently sketched futuristic designs for them on napkins. He also read voraciously, alternating between Chekhov and the latest pharmaceutical study to catch his eye at the UCLA biomedical library, which he entered with a bogus ID scammed at Gold's. His ironies seemed endless. For a guy who seemed outwardly conservative—his closet was filled with chinos and polo shirts—he had a decadent catalog of things that he wanted to try, including a 1945 Château La Fleur-Pétrus and a threesome. (He was willing to sample them separately or together.) What really bound the two men, however, was the idea that Duchaine kept coming back to:

They were at the beginning of something big.

The Olympics were coming to Los Angeles in 1984 and with them a caravan of athletes who would be on the lookout for the latest muscle-building concoctions. They could laugh about which Gold's regulars were trying to follow Arnold into the movies. But five years after the debut of *Pumping Iron*, everyone in L.A. wanted the Schwarzenegger look. More ominously, a new disease that was killing gay men in San Francisco had begun its fatal migration down the Pacific coast. Gay men were turning to steroids to prevent the disease's wasting affect.

Duchaine might not have known as much as Zumpano did about steroids, but he knew enough to understand that, at this moment, in this place, he had stumbled into his future. All the arrows pointed in one direction—to a drug that was almost mystical in its powers, that could turn men into supermen, that could heal the sick, that could make just about anyone feel younger.

And yet, remarkably, steroids didn't have a true constituency. They cut across age and class lines and were undeniably effective, yet they were still subject to whisper campaigns and unflattering propaganda. Steroids needed a champion, a spokesman, a zealot. Duchaine had used them to reinvent himself. Now he wanted to return the favor and reinvent them for America.

One day, he dropped by Zumpano's apartment overcome with excitement. "Jump on, I have something I want to show you," he said.

Zumpano grabbed his knapsack and slid onto the back of the scooter. Once they were underway, Duchaine handed him a page of handwritten notes.

Zumpano started reading.

"We know this will make us a lot of enemies," the notes began. "But although we'll antagonize many of you, we thought we should tell the truth about steroids."

"What's this?" Zumpano asked.

"It's the beginning of the book we're going to write."

A how-to guide for steroid users struck Zumpano as a good idea. He had started researching them to gain a better understanding of his own physiology and already had egg cartons full of files. Why not share his knowledge? The reason for Sunday School was to keep guys from taking the wrong things, or the right things in the wrong doses. Granted, he wasn't a doctor, but he knew as much as any MD he had ever met, especially the ones who preyed on the bodybuilders by trading steroids for sex. Why not put it all in a book? Why not empower guys to make the right decisions?

Duchaine had even bigger ideas. He saw it as a manifesto, a statement of principles regarding life and how to live it. He would be calling on a new generation to drop in and turn on. As they arrived on the pier at Santa Monica, Duchaine turned to Zumpano.

"This is how we're going to be famous," he said.

Zumpano climbed off the back of the scooter and looked at his friend. "You're crazy, you know that, Dan?"

Duchaine wasn't giving up. He read Zumpano a list of words he had picked out for the title. Bible. Muscle. Underground. Anabolic. Zumpano watched the Ferris wheel on the beach turn and tried to put the puzzle pieces together. "What about the *Underground Steroid Handbook*?" he asked.

Being friends with Duchaine was one thing. Being his business partner was another. He started showing up to Zumpano's apartment early in the mornings with bags full of fresh fruit—pomegranates, oranges, and mangos—and would announce, "Time to write."

Over ten feverish days in October 1981, Zumpano worked around the clock, dumping all that he knew onto the creaky keys of an Underwood typewriter. Duchaine picked up the pages each morning, occasionally tweaking text, but mostly leaving his partner alone. When it was finally done, they took it to a friend who had an offset press in his garage and had it typeset into 18 pages, framed by a brown cover of slightly thicker stock. Half how-to-manual, half catalog, their anonymously written manifesto mixed serious discussion with a wit that reflected their rebel mindset.

"We're going to tell you how to keep your doctor happy with your health while you are on steroids," began its authors. "You need protein to make muscles grow, but you need to convince the cell to grow. That's one thing that steroids do." In their introduction, they pointed out that artificial steroids are "those made outside the body," and that they came in two forms: "oral, as a tablet to be swallowed, and injectable, as a liquid to be placed within the muscle." But the real heart of it—what Duchaine called "maybe the most valuable information you'll find in this book"—was the listing of the drugs themselves. Anadrol. Anavar. Bolasterone. Deca-Durabolin. Dianabol. Down the line they went, with 29 drugs in all. Each listing had a review and often a suggested price. ("Anavar doesn't make you all that big, it makes you very strong.") And each, they pointed out, was easily available from the right kind of doctor.

"Most doctors have formed an opinion on steroids, which means they don't like them. Lucky for us though there is a large number of what we call the 'businessman doctor.' These guys are out to hustle a buck .... Look for the young ones just out of medical school. Young doctors have a different morality than then older ones. Many do the standard recreational drugs and are open minded about steroids."

In early 1982, a tiny ad appeared in *Muscle Builder & Power* magazine hawking the *Underground Steroid Handbook for Men and Women*. Checks or money orders for $6, it announced, could be made payable to a company called OEM Media and sent to a P.O. Box in Venice. A few days after the ad appeared, Duchaine visited the mailbox, which was in a small cigar shop on Venice Boulevard. He wasn't sure what he would find, but felt confident that there would be at least a letter or two. A disappointed look crossed his face when he found it empty. As he turned to shuffle out, he mumbled to the counterman, "I hoped we'd have something."

"But you do," the clerk replied, and he handed Duchaine a stack of nearly a hundred envelopes that wouldn't fit in the box.

Duchaine rushed back to the small office that Zumpano kept at Gold's and carefully counted out each check. When they passed $500, they ran into an alley behind Gold's and started kicking a can like kids. Then the budding gurus spent it as fast as it had come in. Zumpano paid off a phone bill that a friend's drunken mother had run up at his apartment. Duchaine bought some clothes— more chinos and polo shirts—and took his partner to lunch at a restaurant owned by a hot new chef, Wolfgang Puck. With what was left, they went on a three-day spending spree. And when they ran out of money, more envelopes were waiting. And more arrived after that. An order for 5,000 books from France, another for 3,000 from Germany. Opening them became such a chore that Zumpano asked his housekeeper to help. By the spring of 1982, they had sold 80,000 books, making nearly a half-million dollars.

At tax time, Zumpano asked Duchaine how much they should declare. Duchaine looked at him disbelievingly. "Taxes? Fuck taxes. Fuck the government." His nose wasn't pressed against the window of Sunday School any longer. He was finally an Arnoldista. And like the rest of them, he had reinvented himself with a new image, one right out of Shakespeare: The Guru of Venice.

PART I

BAND OF BELIEVERS
1981-1992

1

THE GURU OF VENICE

December 11, 1985 - May 10, 1987

Dennis Degan tacked the article from *Sports Illustrated* to his bulletin board and let out a sigh.

As an investigator for the U.S. Food and Drug Administration, Degan had a job that drew snickers from the cops at more glamorous agencies. It involved processing legal actions for field agents who found violations at drug labs or fish factories. But Degan had also begun nosing around the bodybuilding business. And what he found there was turning him into an unlikely soldier in President Ronald Reagan's war on drugs.

During the summer of 1984, Degan was tipped off about a Detroit company that was openly selling steroids without prescriptions, a violation of the 1938 Food, Drug, and Cosmetic Act. After making a few undercover buys, he also learned that it was getting its supply from a mountain of a man named Larry Pacifico. Handsome and wealthy, Pacifico was perhaps the greatest power lifter of all time, having been a nine-time world champion. When Degan confronted him, Pacifico said just enough to make Degan realize that a silent network of steroid dealers existed, and they were using bodybuilding shows as a base of operations. In September 1984, Degan flew to Washington, D.C., and told his bosses he wanted to follow up on the finding. He left with a green light and the makings of a flashy new title: National Steroid Investigation Coordinator.

Two months later, word reached Degan about an arrest in San Diego. An Englishman named Tony Fitton had been stopped at the Mexican border with more than two thousand boxes of Dianabol in his car. Degan recognized the name. Fitton was one of the people whose name had surfaced in the Pacifico investigation. He had worked at an outfit on the campus of Auburn University called The National Strength Research Institute. Its ostensible mission was to hold training seminars for strength coaches, many of whom worked for Division I Bowl caliber teams. But it provided Fitton with a subterranean side business: selling those coaches steroids.

The job of prosecuting Fitton fell to an assistant U.S. Attorney named Phillip Halpern. On December 19, 1984, Degan flew to San Diego to tell Halpern what he knew, and together they were able to build a case that charged Fitton with illegally importing steroids. Fitton pleaded guilty in February 1985 to conspiracy, illegally importing a prohibited substance, and giving false statements. He then jumped bail, forcing agents to trail him through Alabama, New Jersey, and Chicago before he was finally captured, five months later, in Albuquerque, New Mexico.

The *Sports Illustrated* article that Degan had just cut out was about Fitton's sentencing the week before in San Diego federal court. Fitton had been given only five years—a third of what he was eligible to get. With time served, he would be out in a few months.

When Degan took his new job, he knew that he would have a lot of work ahead of him. But he didn't think that work would include convincing the law enforcement community to take the problem seriously.

CARLSBAD, CALIFORNIA
January 1986

Sitting at a local Italian restaurant, Dan Duchaine listened to two friends discuss an enterprise that was going to make them richer than anything they had tried so far.

To his right was David Jenkins, a former Olympic track medalist. Jenkins still had the athletic look that he had carried as a teen in Britain, where he was so popular that he had two nicknames, The Flying Scotsman and The Golden Boy. He had been the youngest to win a 400-meter title, having done so at 19, and anchored Britain's four-man relay team to Olympic silver the next year in Munich. But that was already a lifetime ago for Jenkins. Though he still carried the bearing of a prep school student from his days at Edinburgh Academy, his athletic career was long over. Like so many prodigies who tried to prolong things, he was now 34 and wondering what to do next.

On Duchaine's left was a man who couldn't have been more different than Jenkins. William Dillon had flowing blonde hair, a square jaw, and a more-than-passing resemblance to the pop star Andy Gibb. His six-foot, 200-pound frame had won him a Mr. Collegiate Illinois bodybuilding title while he was studying mechanical engineering at Southern Illinois University. As soon as he graduated, he took a job in Los Angeles, where he went to work for the aerospace division of Hughes Aircraft. Lately, he had made a second home for himself at Gold's.

All three men in the restaurant that January day had experience with steroids. Jenkins came across his knowledge in 1975, when he was preparing for the Montreal Olympic games. He loaded up on a cycle, then stopped a few weeks before the competition to ensure that he wouldn't be caught. Unfortunately for him, the drugs didn't help. He failed to get a medal and was an afterthought four years later, when he made one last stab at Olympic glory in Moscow.

Dillon, meanwhile, had learned all he needed about steroids at Gold's, where he worked out on the same machines as Michael Landon, who was starring in *Highway to Heaven*, and Carl Weathers, who had just reprised his role as Apollo Creed in *Rocky IV*. One day, a workout partner at the gym offered Dillon a cycle of Sustanon 250 and the results were so remarkable that he had to have more. He soon started dealing, and quickly worked his way up the supply ladder to Duchaine, who was wholesaling steroids from his home. Within six months, Dillon had become Duchaine's largest customer. But there was always room to get bigger, and Jenkins had invited them to dinner on this balmy January evening to explain how.

The FDA had just sent a letter to America's major drug makers, asking them to stop selling steroids that lacked any legitimate medical application. The move was partly a reaction to the college sports scandals of the past year—including the one involving Fitton— but it had a strange side effect. Overnight, the supply of several of America's most popular steroids, including Dianabol, dried up. "I think I have someone in Mexico who can make Dianabol," Jenkins said. "If my guy can make it, can you guys sell it?"

With Dillon's head for business, and Duchaine's contacts in the drug world, they had no doubts. "Think about it, we'll be making our own steroids," Duchaine said, eyes alight with thoughts of what seemed a thrilling new adventure, like skydiving or drag racing, but with an international element of danger. He didn't think twice about breaking the law. In a recent issue of *Sports Illustrated*, Fitton had been described as "perhaps the largest single steroid dealer in the world," yet he would probably wind up doing less than a year in a minimum-security federal work camp. "No one goes to jail for a long time for this," Duchaine said, taking another step away from the mainstream.

TIJUANA, MEXICO
February 1986

David Jenkins walked into the swank Fiesta Americana hotel and took the elevator up to the fourth floor, where he found the head-quarters of Laboratorios Milanos and its president, Juan Macklis.

Jenkins had come to know Macklis quite by accident. He had been at a supplement convention, trying to figure out how to break into the business, when he noticed a Laboratorios Milanos booth selling tamper-proof packaging. Before he knew it, he was talking with Macklis about other things that his company could supply, namely steroids.

A circumspect man who had powerful friends in Mexico—it was said he had important allies in the country's notoriously corrupt police department—Macklis controlled a pharmaceutical factory two miles away. It was pink and yellow, and heavily fortified by armed guards. As they got down to business, Jenkins wanted to know how much Macklis would charge him for 100 tablets of Dianabol. Macklis told Jenkins that he'd charge $1.45, even though it only cost him half of that to make it. Jenkins was only too happy to say yes as he and his new partners were going to sell them for even more than that. Selling on the street, they could get $35 for one of the bottles.

Three months later, Jenkins reconvened with his partners at a restaurant near a health food company he had started in Carlsbad. After they talked about sports and politics, Jenkins nodded to Dillon, who handed over a bag with $30,000 in it. In return, Jenkins slid a set of directions across the table, along with a room key. When dessert was finished, Duchaine and Dillon said goodbye and followed the directions to the Allstar Inn, where they found suitcases on the bed packed with steroids.

These pills were designed to blow away the competition. Dillon came up with the idea of counterfeiting European pharmaceutical labels so their customers would think they were getting top-shelf stuff with dosages higher than anything else on the street. Opening up one case, Duchaine let out a slow whistle. "I'd be fooled by these," he said.

Throughout the spring, their operation grew. The quintet hadn't so much replaced Fitton in the steroid underground as turned him into an afterthought. So much money was coming in that it was a struggle to spend it all. Dillon quit his job at Hughes and quietly started investing. He bought a stake in a Venice restaurant and a Gold's Gym in San Diego, and eyed a farm in Illinois that he thought he might soon retire to with his wife. Duchaine, however, kept crossing things off his list of things that he wanted to try. A few weeks earlier, Dillon had shown up at the red-brick home that Duchaine leased by the Venice boardwalk and found a Maserati parked outside; Duchaine had rented it for the day for a drive up the coast. Then there was the thousand-dollar bottle of wine sitting in Duchaine's kitchen. "Open it," he said. "Haven't you ever wondered what wine like that tastes like?"

Since he was easily bored, Duchaine satisfied most of his cravings after just one try. But there was one he couldn't drop—a morphine substitute called Nubain. To bodybuilders who came to him for advice, he enthused about its ability to take the edge off aches and pains that came from overtraining. But Nubain also took the edge off what few inhibitions the 34-year-old guru had left. While in its throes, he had a fling with one of his ex-wife's acquaintances on a houseboat and promptly started seeing her. Her openness to bisexuality thrilled him and he paid $5,000 for them to join a sex club. After all those years in the gym, his body had finally reached a kind of mid-30s zenith, lean and tanned and rippling in all the right places. Even his hair was cooperating; it was full and black and dramatic when combed back. With more money than he needed, he was free to disappear into the character he had invented for himself—the one that Nubain freed him to imagine in deeper and darker hues, aided by a growing list of friends and business partners who seemed like they were from a B movie: porn stars, mobsters, rogue cops. His home may have had a white picket fence around it, but that was as close as Dan Duchaine was getting to Middle America.

With a lifestyle like that, it was inevitable that law enforcement would start looking into his affairs. When Mike Zumpano came back to Venice for a visit in the early spring, he went for a drive with Duchaine—the two had formally dissolved their business arrangement three years earlier so Zumpano could open a vitamin and supplement company—and noticed his old partner looking in his rearview mirror.

"What's going on?" he asked.

"I think we're being followed," Duchaine replied.

Soon after, Duchaine went to a store where he kept a P.O. Box and nodded to the owner. He was met by a grim look. When the owner held up his hands, he saw why. To signal that the feds were watching, the man had written three letters on his knuckles: F-B-I.

That night, Duchaine called Dillon and told him to move whatever steroids he had on hand out of his house. The feds were on their trail.

Dillon, meanwhile, had picked up his own tail. As he zipped through Venice on his scooter, he began to notice a beige sedan following him, and not always successfully. On one trip, the sedan got stuck in an alley and Dillon sped around the block to come up behind it. Without saying a word, he gave a slight wave to the men in suits in the front seat.

Eventually, LAPD officers raided his house along with one that belonged to an acquaintance whom he had begun paying to store and ship his drugs. In a fortunate fluke, Dillon had removed $75,000 from his dresser that morning and put it in the trunk of his scooter—a place the cops never searched. But they had found something even more incriminating in his friend's garage: bogus prescription steroid labels.

Sitting in his friend's lawn chair, Dillon acted nonchalant as the LAPD asked him about the labels. He kept his cool, trying to convince the cops that he was a small-time operator. And to Dillon's relief, they appeared to believe him. As soon as they left, he grabbed a bulky new device he had bought—something called a cell phone—and dialed Duchaine. "It's gotten too hot here," he said. "I'm getting out."

"Just as well," Duchaine told his friend. "If it gets nasty, you won't be good at it."

SAN DIEGO
December 1986

William Dillon moved south to San Diego, hoping to escape the attention of the cops. But that proved easier said than done. The persuasive David Jenkins kept after him, trying to lure him back into the fold. Jenkins was complaining that he hadn't been able to replace the customers they had lost when Dillon pulled out. If Dillon would just introduce those customers directly to Jenkins— just make a few calls—he could have 10 percent of the profits, right off the top. How could he say no?

The problem was that one of his first deals for Jenkins had gone horribly wrong, as one of their best customers had gotten ripped off by a prospective client and had hired a hit man to get even. The client had wound up running to the cops and telling all he knew about the drug ring. Soon Dennis Degan was being called into the case and learning, for the first time, that William Dillon and Dan Duchaine were partners.

What the ripped-off client couldn't say was where Dillon and Duchaine were getting their steroids. Who was the mysterious Mr. X?

That question led Degan to fly to San Diego to set up surveillance outside Dillon's Gold's Gym. But after two weeks of watching Dillon's comings and goings, and taking photos of the gym's clientele, the fed was still no closer to an answer. What he needed was someone on the inside. For help he turned to the man whose home he had raided two years before, the wealthy champion power lifter Larry Pacifico.

If there was a single trait that made Pacifico stand out, it was that he was virtually impossible not to like. Even Degan found him irrepressibly charming. But he had another trait that was even more useful. The 40-year-old Pacifico was practical. After he was charged with receiving steroids from the Netherlands in the summer of 1986, he decided to salvage what he could by cooperating with the feds. Pacifico offered to help Degan by calling Toivol Mansen, a Florida bodybuilder who once worked for him at his spa, with a phony story: Pacifico had an armed guard who wanted to make a large purchase of steroids. Could Mansen help out?

Eager to help his old boss, Mansen agreed to meet the newcomer in Miami. Pacifico's "guard" was really an undercover U.S. Customs Department agent who had been carefully screened by Degan. Mansen received him warmly. Any friend of Larry Pacifico, he said, was a friend of his. Mansen then opened up about a deal that he was working on, a big steroid buy in which he was personally investing $60,000. Mansen said that he thought there was room for others and the undercover agent brightened. Mansen agreed to bring him to meet Dillon, the brains behind the buy.

Two days later, at a hotel near Sea World, Dillon was happy to embrace a moneyed friend of Pacifico's. In great and injudicious detail, he talked about Jenkins and the pipeline they had to Mexico, and how the upcoming buy would work. The undercover agent had been instructed to find out as much as he could without actually spending any of the government's money. So he laid a trap. Before he actually invested anything, he said, he would need to see how the operation worked. Dillon and Mansen agreed that this made sense and proposed that the newcomer accompany Mansen on a warm-up buy before he spent his own cash.

Early in the morning of March 20, 1987, Mansen picked up the undercover agent and drove to the San Diego border. From there they crossed into Tijuana on foot and walked to the Hotel Fiesta. Waiting for them in room 408 was Jenkins—the man who was still only known to law enforcement as the mysterious Mr. X.

The cautious Jenkins rose from his breakfast and conducted the day's first piece of business. He accepted roughly $200,000 from Mansen and in return handed over the keys to a truck that was parked across the border and filled with steroids that had been smuggled separately. Mansen thanked him and left, taking his companion back to the San Diego side of the border, where they found the truck and unloaded it.

Now that Jenkins had proven himself reliable, the next step was to make the bigger buy.

For that, Mansen and his undercover investor went to a safety-deposit box in San Ysidro, where Degan had arranged for $250,000 in cash to be placed. The agent loaded it into a duffel bag stamped with a Gold's Gym logo, and watched as Mansen added another $120,000 representing his own money and the investments of the others in Dillon's group. Once the bag was stuffed, they set out for their second trip of the morning across the border.

This time, however, Degan made sure that things wouldn't go as smoothly. He'd arranged for customs officers to stop the pair and ask if they were taking more than $10,000 into Mexico. When they replied no, the officers would ask for the bag to be opened.

The scheme went off exactly as planned. As the agent got cuffed, he screamed at Mansen as if he were furious, saying there would be hell to pay. Mansen, meanwhile, was led to a small office where he was held for questioning. Several hours later, he was released, but not before word had hit the street that the whole thing had been a rip-off planned by Dillon.

That wasn't true, of course, but it had the benefit of turning up the heat on Dillon. As his former friends demanded their money,

Dillon stayed in his house, afraid to go out. The final straw came when he got a call from a hit man whom he knew from Gold's. The hit man said that a contract was out on Dillon's life and he intended to do the job.

Dillon hung up the phone and realized Dan Duchaine was right. He wasn't good when things got nasty. The next day, Dillon hired an attorney who called Phillip Halpern. "My client would like to make a deal," the lawyer told the federal prosecutor.

SAN DIEGO
May 10, 1987

William Dillon picked up the phone in the U.S. Attorney's Office and dialed Dan Duchaine's phone number. When Duchaine answered, Dillon was surprised to find him mired in a depression. Dillon had since pleaded guilty to conspiracy and illegal importation and distribution of steroids. (David Jenkins, meanwhile, pleaded guilty to possessing mislabeled steroids for sale, among other charges.) It had been months since they had spoken, and the Dan he knew—the happy-go-lucky, fiercely independent guy—now sounded sullen. Dillon wondered whether it was really Dan he was hearing, or someone lost in a Nubain haze.

A few months earlier, Duchaine had decided he needed a break from Venice. Hell, a break from the whole drug-dealing life. For a change of pace, he accepted an invitation from his old partner, Mike Zumpano, to move up north and work at the vitamin company Zumpano now owned. But it didn't go well. Duchaine was no more suited for a desk job than he was for life on a fishing trawler. One morning, he started throwing chairs in the middle of Zumpano's office, raving, "Life is so fucked up, we should all be dead." Once Zumpano was able to calm him down, they retired to the lunchroom.

"What's wrong, Dan?" he asked.

Duchaine buried his head in his hands and started crying. "It's the Nubain, Mike," he said. "I'm hooked. Shit, I'm taking 20 valiums a day and Halcion, too."

It was getting harder for Duchaine to tell whether he was being paranoid or just keenly observant. He obsessed about a dish atop a neighboring apartment building that he was sure had been put there by the feds to listen to his conversations. From his living room, he kept staring at a boat that bobbed along the inland waterway, positive that FBI agents were inside of it, snapping long-range pictures.

Oddly, he didn't think twice when William Dillon called him out of the blue. "How've you been, William?" he said softly into the receiver.

"I've been on edge, pretty much," Dillon replied.

Duchaine admitted that he was, too, then tried to sound supportive. "I don't think you have any worry from the government. If they wanted to do anything, it would have been done."

Anyway, Duchaine said, it was a good time to get out of the business. What he had started five years ago with the *Underground Steroid Handbook* was spiraling out of his control.

"I went out and bought all the things I wanted to buy," he said. "But then I really got tired of them. Now that I bought all my toys, I really have nothing I really want to go out and buy."

"It's weird," Dillon said, steering the conversation back to what the prosecutors wanted to know about. "What started off innocent ... it just turned into a monster."

Duchaine murmured his agreement. Then he said something that struck Dillon as very sad.

"You really can't trust anything from the underground anymore."

2

"ZEE CODES, ZEY ARE MISSING"

May 1988 - March 1, 1989

Don Catlin drove from his West Los Angeles laboratory to the Santa Monica pier, where he slipped on a pair of rollerblades so he could skate onto Venice Beach. The midmorning constitutional was more than a way to ease the pressures of a demanding job. It was a way for him to do that job.

The 49-year-old doctor was a natural sleuth. In years past, he had occasionally grabbed a seat by the weight racks by Muscle Beach and stared out at the Pacific, trying not to be obvious about eavesdropping on the bodybuilders who were flexing on weight benches. Tall and unassuming, there was nothing in Catlin's look—a UCLA T-shirt and baggy shorts—to suggest that the horizon he was looking over was filled with intrigue.

A New Englander who had received an undergraduate diploma from Yale and his medical degree from the University of Rochester, Catlin had made a name for himself as a young doctor by helping to wean Vietnam veterans off their heroin and morphine addictions. His work at Walter Reed Army Medical Center in Washington, D.C., led to a teaching and research position in pharmacology at the UCLA Medical School. That put him on a relatively short list of available local experts when the International Olympic Committee needed someone to oversee a drug-testing lab for the 1984 Summer Games. At first, he told his suitors that they had the wrong man. What did he know about sports, much less boutique ones like archery? But the IOC executives were persuasive. Catlin envisioned a 1000-square-foot lab on the grounds of UCLA filled with the latest equipment. He couldn't refuse.

It didn't take long for the doctor to be thrown into the maw. On a humid August night in 1983, an incident unfolded in Caracas, Venezuela, where the Pan American Games were being held. Acting on a tip, police fanned out across the city, raiding athletes' dorms in search of performance-enhancing drugs. By the end of the investigation, 19 competitors from ten nations had been disqualified from the games. In the panic that ensued, several Americans from track and field slipped out unnoticed by catching a late-night flight.

Media reports about the incident embarrassed the leadership of the U.S. Olympic Committee, which promptly went into emergency session. A week later, it emerged with a new plan designed to show it was taking the drug issue seriously. Its athletes would be asked to submit to random testing, which Catlin would then analyze. If they tested positive, they would receive counseling, but the results would be kept confidential.

Catlin saw the policy for what it was: a PR stunt. Since the athletes knew there was no punishment, they would simply experiment with performance-enhancing drugs until they could determine the maximum amount of drugs that would not trigger a positive test. Far from deterring cheating, the USOC had put itself, and Catlin, in bed with the perpetrators.

The 1984 Olympic Games opened on Saturday, July 28, in an atmosphere of enormous political tension. The Soviets were boycotting the games to protest the Reagan Administration's cold war policies. And instead of trying to lower the political thermostat, the Los Angeles organizing committee produced an over-the-top, flag-draped Hollywood pageant at the opening ceremonies. Four miles away in his lab, Catlin went to work.

Over the next two weeks, he would analyze 1,507 samples and find 12 confirmed positives.[1] But the biggest bang was reserved for the final weekend, when all eyes were on Carl Lewis, who was trying to tie Jesse Owens's 1936 record of four gold medals in track & field in a single Olympics.

Grim-faced couriers dumped scores of new samples on his lab, forcing Catlin and his staff to work around the clock to meet the demand. It wasn't until Wednesday, August 15th—after Lewis succeeded in matching Owens's record and the Olympic flame was extinguished—that he handed his final results to Prince Alexandre de Mérode of Belgium, the chairman of the IOC's Medical Commission. Catlin couldn't say to whom the samples belonged because only numbers identified them; the Prince kept the master list that matched them to names. All he knew was that he had turned up nine more positives.

With most of the press packing up, Catlin wondered whether his findings would ever get reported. The Games had surpassed *Roots*, Alex Haley's landmark miniseries, as the highest-rated TV event on ABC, and Ronald Reagan, who opened the Games, was getting ready to welcome the medal winners to the White House. The next day, de Mérode walked into Catlin's office with news that assured the answer would be no.

"Zee safe where I put zee results eez gone," de Mérode said. Overnight, someone had moved the safe to a storage facility in

---

1 They belonged to, among others, a Swedish wrestler, a Finnish long-distance runner, a Greek javelin thrower, weightlifters from Lebanon and Algeria, an Icelandic discus thrower, and an Italian hammer thrower.

Culver City. When he went to look inside, the codes weren't there. "Zee codes, zey are missing," he said.

The doctor couldn't believe it. His results were meaningless without the codes. But what could he do? Exhausted, Catlin closed down his lab and returned to teaching, letting the mystery of the missing list—and the thief who took it—weigh on him.

Was there an American star among the positives?

Were the L.A. Games rigged in advance?

A year later, when the USOC approached him to ask if he would be interested in restarting the lab on a full-time basis, Catlin decided that he couldn't leave the adventure that he had started. He submitted a detailed proposal that was ultimately approved, officially making him America's chief Olympic steroid hunter. By 1988, his work had earned him a spot on the IOC's Medical Commission as well.

Now, as he bladed along the Venice boardwalk, he thought about the trip he would soon be taking to Seoul, South Korea, where the Summer Games would be held. What new drug scandal, he wondered, would await him there?

It was a question that a doctor much like Catlin had asked 30 years earlier, when the drug revolution in American sports was just getting underway.

OLNEY, MARYLAND

Spring 1959

To the senior citizens of Olney, Maryland, John Ziegler was an affable country doctor. He helped them strengthen their brittle bones and atrophied muscles with weights, much how he had rebuilt his own after the war. At Snuffy's, a local bar with dirt floors, the regulars didn't even know he was a doctor. All they knew was that their friend, Big John, had a restless, imaginative intellect, and when a few bourbons got mixed in, his ideas came spilling out loudly and profanely. He had hoped to become a brain surgeon, but had been prevented by his war injuries. So he became a medical bon vivant, collecting an MD while studying everything from nuclear medicine to hypnosis, and holding a weekly salon in his living room, where his suburban Washington guests ranged from White House staffers to Marine generals and astrophysicists.

In the summer of 1959, Ziegler's most intense curiosity was reserved for how the body grew muscle. Medical investigators, he knew, had tried to unlock the keys to masculinity as early as the 18th century. But it took another hundred years for someone to extend the inquiries to athletics. In 1894, Austrian physiologist Oskar Zoth and his partner Fritz Pregl, a physician who went on to win the Nobel Prize for chemistry in 1923, injected themselves with an extract from bulls' testicles. While the pair reported feeling stronger, there is no evidence that the extract had any true physical effect. Two years later, Zoth wrote a paper on the study, concluding prophetically: "the training of athletes offers an opportunity for further research, and for a practical assessment of our experimental results."

Soon, others were taking up the challenge. In 1910, a German physiologist injected sperm into dogs to see if it stopped them from tiring when they ran on a treadmill. He achieved no notable success. But 30 years later, Third Reich scientists succeeded in isolating the male sex hormone and were reportedly giving shots of synthesized testosterone to Adolf Hitler.

Of course, the Nazis were trying to breed a master race, not make better athletes. (Singular achievement was anathema to the Fascist philosophy—as was drug and alcohol use.) But their interest in another hormone, adrenaline, would help future researchers to do just that. In one fateful experiment, Nazi researchers broke the leg of a frog and then covered it with a splint, hoping to study the pace of its atrophy. The frog surprised them, however, by fighting its splint until the damaged leg had more muscle than the unbroken one.

Ziegler became aware of the underground research into hormones when he traveled to Europe in 1954, as an advisor to the U.S. weightlifting team. Having caught sight of Russian athletes using catheters to urinate, Ziegler asked a Russian physician whom he had met at a beer hall about it. The doctor confessed that his coaches were extending the work of the Nazis by injecting their athletes with straight testosterone.

When he returned to America, Ziegler began his own experiments and hit upon a formula for what he would later call a "kinder, gentler" synthetic testosterone. His aim was to bombard "receptor" cells in the muscles with a compound that would help them absorb protein and grow. The key was to do it while limiting the androgenic side effects, such as higher blood pressure and cholesterol levels, which, in women, can also lead to facial hair and deeper voices. Ziegler achieved it with a synthetic compound called methandrostenolone. In 1958, a New Jersey drug company bought it for $100 and named the result Dianabol.

The pill clearly had wonderfully curative powers. It reversed the effects of osteoporosis in some elderly patients. And in burn victims it seemed to help regrow skin. But soon Ziegler was eager to try it on healthier subjects.

Ziegler ultimately worked with a young lifter named Billy March, who visited his home one day in 1959. "I want you to take two of these a day between meals," Ziegler said, handing March two Dianabol tablets. March accepted the pills and swallowed them nervously.

It was a crucial step in a nascent athletic cold war.

Thanks in part to Ziegler's little pink pills, March began out-lifting everyone in America. In 1963, he placed third in the world championships in Budapest. His exploits were breathlessly reported in the pages of *Strength & Health* magazine. Meanwhile, Ziegler was continuing his work on the chemical front. By early 1963, he had developed an injectable steroid called Winstrol that used an oil base to carry the testosterone directly to the muscle. In a letter dated February 25, 1963, J.R. Lucas, an executive from Winthrop Laboratories in Baltimore, encouraged him to expand those tests. Enthusing about "your plans" to branch into football, Lucas, the manager of the company's Eastern Division Medical Research, wrote:

> In addition to the Chicago Bears, which you mentioned to me, it might be easy to set up a similar study with the Washington Redskins, possibly through Coach Bill McPeak. Another possible place has occurred to us. A study like this might be set up in one of the Marine basic training camps to see if the administration of Winstrol would speed up the physical fitness program ....
>
> I am planning to go down to Annapolis shortly and will talk over the question of a similar study with the football coach down there.

But soon Ziegler was tempering his enthusiasm for drugs. Thanks to the arrival of Dianabol on the West Coast, bodybuilders there were posting astounding lifts. (According to one story, the biggest names all gathered in a Mafia-like sit-down, agreeing that competitors wouldn't be allowed to take more than two tablets a day.) In Olney, Ziegler's phone was ringing off the hook. Some days, his driveway wasn't big enough for all the cars that wanted to park in it.

He finally had enough when he learned that lifters he had advised were taking doses as high as 200 milligrams a week—up to ten times Ziegler's recommendation. Rising from his seat, he yelled to one friend, "If those simple-minded shits won't follow my advice, I won't write any more prescriptions. Don't they know I'm the doctor?"

By January 1967, Ziegler had tired of trying to counsel a generation that saw him as an aging crank. As Doctor Dianabol, he had changed the rules of weightlifting. Now it was time to stay in Olney and watch the world he had created spin on its own.

PADUA, ITALY

June 13, 1988

Charlie Francis couldn't believe he was breaking up with someone he had nearly been married to for the last dozen years. If it had been a woman, he would have known what to say. But this was Ben Johnson, the once scrawny 15-year-old boy he had turned into the fastest man in the world.

Johnson was exquisitely sensitive when it came to his body. He claimed he could feel when he was a tenth of a second slower than he should be on the track. He was also sensitive about loyalty. And since he had just set the world 100-meter record in Rome the prior fall, he had been brooding that Francis was taking him for granted.

Things came to a head at the start of 1988's outdoor season when Johnson re-injured his hamstring. Instead of rehabbing with Francis, he traveled to the Caribbean island of St. Kitt's to do it on his own and show Francis who was really in control.

Francis knew from experience how easy it was for an athlete to destroy his body by thinking he knew best. And the move left him in a rage. Well, then go to hell, Francis said. If you think you know better than me, you're on your own.

Now, after not talking to each other for a month, they were crossing paths again in Padua, Italy, where Johnson was contractually obligated to attend a meet. "I don't know how we can work together if you won't listen to me," Francis told him.

"Then I guess we can't," Johnson shot back.

Francis wasn't used to sprinters walking out on him, especially not three months before the Olympic Games in Seoul. His track club, Mazda Optimists, was the subject of intense gossip among rival coaches. They were circulating rumors—hurtful and devastating rumors—that he was giving drugs to his sprinters. Of course, those rumors also happened to be true.

He could only fend them off so long as his group stuck together. But now, Ben Johnson was off the reservation.

Things had been so much easier for Francis in the early 1970s, when he was the world's fifth-ranked sprinter and was studying history on a scholarship to Stanford University. He was so highly regarded that he was selected to represent Canada at the Munich Olympics. It was there that he saw a couple of sprinters openly pop pink Dianabol tablets—which wouldn't be banned by the IOC until 1975—and figured, what the hell, he might as well too. Using himself as a kind of lab, he learned all he could about the drugs. Soon he came to the conclusion that a sprinter at the peak of his or her form could gain roughly a meter advantage in a 100-meter dash.

That knowledge came a little late to do much good for Francis's running career. He retired in 1974 and then disappeared from the scene to sell insurance. It wasn't until a friend convinced him that he should try part-time coaching that he realized he had a talent for it. Francis was demanding, to be sure. And, yes, he had a temper. But he stood by his sprinters, often spending what little money he had on food or clothes for them. Back then, Eddie Johnson, Ben's older brother, looked to be the promising one. Ben, the fifth of six children, was just a gawky 93-pounder who hung around the track at York University in Toronto, where Francis coached. During their first summer together, Ben put on six inches and 43 pounds, quickly rising to become one of Francis's most exciting and durable sprinters. By the early 1980s, he was well known in Canada. But everywhere else in the track world, the talk was about Carl Lewis, the New Jersey sensation with a flattop haircut.

In September 1981, Francis sat down with his young charge and told him a few facts of pharmaceutical life. If Ben wanted to chase Carl Lewis on the world stage, he said, leaning in to make his point, he would have to make a decision about how far he was willing to go.

Under Francis's watchful eye, the 19-year-old Johnson started taking five-milligram doses of Dianabol daily over three-week on-off cycles, then stepped up to the milder but longer-lasting stanozolol. But as of late, Johnson was still having trouble breaking through the magical 10.0-second mark. So before the 1984 Games, Francis visited an L.A. doctor who specialized in exploiting the loopholes in the Olympics drug-testing policy. He delivered Francis a new shopping list, which included human growth hormone and a trio of amino acids that boosted the body's natural hormonal production. Next, Francis brought the list to a Toronto doctor he knew and had three other compounds added to it: oral Dianabol, injectable vitamin B-12, and small doses of inosine, a non-steroidal anabolic.

It was an extraordinary collection of drugs. And with them, Johnson won the bronze medal at the 1984 Games in Los Angeles. He only failed to beat Lewis in the 100-meter final because he cramped up late.

After the 1984 Olympics, Francis started researching new combinations. His Toronto contact suggested that Johnson use injectable Dianabol and, later, a milky-white cousin of stanozolol called furazabol. Francis tried it himself and proclaimed it wonderful; he personally went from bench-pressing 200 pounds to nearly twice that. Johnson loved it, too. With furazabol coursing through his system, he surged into second place in the 1985 standings and twice beat Lewis in 1986.

By 1987, Johnson seemed unstoppable. He ran 44 races in the outdoor season and beat Lewis three more times, including a race in Rome in which he won with a 9.83-second time—shattering the previous world record by a full tenth of a second. The media finally began paying attention to the quiet Jamaican-born sprinter. "He would compress all the anger from all the slights into the heart of his race, into his start," *Sports Illustrated* rhapsodized. "And it would only be afterward, after Rome, after the detonation, that we would begin to suspect what pressures were contained in the vessel that is Ben Johnson."

Lewis, meanwhile, also had suspicions about what was inside Johnson. When they lined up beside one another in Rome, he thought Ben's eyes looked sickly yellow, a sure sign of steroid use. "If I were taking drugs, I could do a 9.80 right away," the exasperated American told Britain's ITV after the Rome race. Then he added, "Just like him." Fearing a lawsuit, the producers left that sound bite on the cutting room floor.

Johnson shrugged off the remark. He was driving around Toronto in a Porsche and juggling several women. "No one gets tested more than me," he told *The Toronto Star*. "If I was losing, I don't think Lewis or anybody else would keep talking about stupid drugs."

But Francis couldn't afford to be so cavalier. Forget Lewis. He had to watch his back in his own country. The doctor who had been advising them in Toronto was getting too big for his britches, trying to convince Johnson that he knew better than Francis how to run. The doctor was also talking too much for anyone's good. He had told another Canadian Olympian that Francis was mismanaging the steroid doses that he had recommended. Word of his athletes' usage reached a rival coach, who fired off a memo to the Canadian Track & Field Association. Given the explosiveness of the allegation, the memo was remarkably restrained. It merely asked that Francis reassure everyone in the group that his methods conformed to the "existing rules." The timely intervention of powerful friends on the group's board allowed Francis not even to admit that much. But the wagons were circling.

Considering the climate, Francis had good reason not to want Johnson out of his sight. It was especially worrisome that Johnson had decided to rehabilitate his strained hamstring on the island of St. Kitt's, where his contact for prescriptions, Dr. Jamie Astaphan, had moved his medical practice. Francis tried to explain when they met at Johnson's hotel in Italy. They were in a critical phase, he said. They needed to close ranks, not have a hanger-on like Astaphan come between them. But Johnson didn't want to hear it.

Well, let Johnson go then, Francis told himself, embittered. He would quickly see that drugs without proper coaching wouldn't do a damned thing.

While Francis continued on through Europe with the rest of his club, Johnson cooled out in St. Kitt's. But he wasn't able to stay there for long. On June 27, Lewis electrified fans in Paris by running a wind-aided time of 9.95 seconds in the 100-meter final. Afterward, Lewis couldn't help but tweak his absent rival.

"The most important thing is that I am running well and he's not running at all," Lewis said. "I hope he gets healthy and has a good season because I intend to."

The next day, *The Toronto Star* did more to get Johnson back together with Francis than anyone. "Big Ben, Coach Must Reconcile or Gold Is Lost," read the headline.

Soon thereafter, a mutual friend arranged to have them meet at his house. "You can't let Carl do this," Francis said.

Ben nodded. After Lewis's performance, they both knew what they needed to do.

SEOUL, SOUTH KOREA
September 24, 1988

The half hour before a big race was always the worst for Charlie Francis. He had naturally high blood pressure. The trick was keeping it low while he waited for the race to start. He found a tunnel by the finish line and ducked into it, trying to measure his breathing.

After a little while, he saw Ben Johnson make his way toward Lane 6. Standing in the finish line tunnel and listening to his own breathing, Francis prayed he had done enough to get Johnson ready to beat Lewis. On August 24, he had called Johnson to his apartment and injected him with furazabol. Four days later, Dr. Astaphan administered another two shots before the team boarded a plane for Korea. They were close to the cut-off line and they knew it. Ideally, they would have stopped the cycle at least a month before a competition. But nothing about these circumstances was ideal. Astaphan was also nervous enough to give Johnson a dose of Moduret, a diuretic that would help pass the steroids through his system more quickly. All they could do now was hope.

When the starter's pistol fired at 1:30 p.m., Johnson was slower out of the blocks than he had been in Rome. But he was still quicker than Lewis. His left hand led him to a leap that turned into more than a foot-long advantage at the 10-meter mark. Seventy thousand people stood in Olympic Stadium, waiting to see Lewis's answer. But, remarkably, there was none. Instead, Johnson was the one who continued to upshift. With his superior muscles manufacturing speed, he ramped up to an incredible 5.02 strides a second at the 40-meter mark. Stealing a look Johnson's way, Lewis pumped methodically, no desperation evident in his beautiful form. By the 60-meter mark, he had succeeded in reaching Johnson's top speed of 12.1 meters a second. But the damage was done. With 15 meters to go, Johnson was so far ahead that he stopped pumping his arms and still glided to a world record 9.79 time.

Francis ran through the cheering throng to get down to Johnson, who had since grabbed a Canadian flag in exhausted delight. There was just one more formality before it all became official, one they had gone through 29 times in the last two years without incident. Ben just had to give a urine sample.

SEOUL, SOUTH KOREA
September 25, 1988

Don Catlin settled into dinner with Robert Dugal, an old friend who had supervised the drug-testing operation at the 1976 Olympics. As a member of the IOC's Medical Commission, Dugal was among the handful of experts overseeing the drug-testing lab in Seoul, and since Catlin was also there as a member of the IOC's medical staff, the two ate together almost every night. They chose the Italian team's hotel because Alitalia flew in fresh pasta daily, and everyone in the Olympic village knew it was where you could find the best food.

After they ordered, Dugal took a piece of paper from his briefcase and slid it over to Catlin. In a thick French-Canadian accent, he said, "Don, tell me what you think of this." Catlin glanced at the page, where two intersecting lines formed a right angle, across which ranged a series of peaks and valleys. To the untrained eye, it looked like the result of a lie detector test, and in some respects, it was.

Catlin immediately recognized it as the result of a test from a gas-chromatography/mass spectrometry machine. Small samples of urine got fed into the machine and heated up to a maximum of 356 degrees, until the liquid turned into a gas. The gas was driven into a coiled chamber, where it was broken down and separated into individual components. After that, each was measured for its mass and molecular makeup. Because steroids leave molecular markers when the body absorbs them, an experienced GC/MS reader could recognize the presence of certain steroids by the peaks on the readout. To Catlin, it wasn't even a question. The athlete whose sample he was staring at had used stanozolol.

"Who is this for?" he asked.

Dugal took a sip of wine before answering indirectly. "All I can tell you is that America is going to win another gold medal."

"It's Ben Johnson?" Catlin asked, losing his breath.

At 7:30 the next morning, Francis was jolted awake by a knock on his dorm room door. According to Olympic rules, a positive drug test had to be confirmed by a second test, which is administered on an extract from the original sample. For the so-called B-test, athletes or their coaches or representatives can be present to witness it. When Francis opened his door, a manager for Canada's track team was anxiously waiting. "We've got to get over to the medical commission," he said. "Ben's tested positive."

Francis tried to absorb the news. It wasn't that Johnson wasn't guilty. It's that the drug testers shouldn't have been able to prove it. The GC/MS machine was only as smart as the people operating it. In other words, it only looked for compounds that it was programmed to seek out. And it wasn't supposed to recognize furazabol, the steroid that Johnson had been using.

Still in a daze, Francis collected his things, joined up with members of the Canadian delegation, and made his way to Dugal's testing lab downtown, followed a short time later by Johnson. At a hearing later that evening, the Canadian delegation tried to press the case that Johnson's postrace samples—the B-test had also come up positive—had been the victim of sabotage. But it didn't work. At 1 a.m., the word reached Francis that their appeal had been rejected. Soon thereafter, Johnson handed over his medal to Olympic authorities and caught a flight back to Toronto.

On the way to his own flight, Francis tried to figure out what the hell had happened to them. If Ben was set up, someone had done a masterful job. He imagined Lewis being handed the gold medal that Johnson had won and it made him dizzy. Sure, he and Johnson had been guilty of doping. And, yes, they had gotten caught. But they had been caught for the wrong thing. And that was what irked him.

As the jet left Seoul behind, Francis couldn't help but feel he was the one who had been cheated.

BAY STREET, TORONTO
March 1, 1989

Charlie Francis cringed at the man selling T-shirts outside the downtown Toronto office building. On one side of the shirt was Ben Johnson's face. On the other were the words, "I didn't do it." Oh yes you did, he thought. And now he was going to tell the national commission of inquiry that had been set up to investigate them exactly how.

By issuing a public denial in the days after Seoul, Francis had bought himself a little time. But not much. Reporters camped out outside his Toronto apartment, forcing him to move to a hotel with his fiancée. His mother had even been tracked down in the cancer ward of a local hospital and asked for comment about her infamous son. He went into seclusion, knowing that it wouldn't be long before the national committee of inquiry, headed by an august judge named Charles Dubin, came with a subpoena for him.

The top female sprinter in his Optimist club had already handed its investigators five years' worth of diaries that chronicled her drug usage. The entries were eye-opening in their matter-of-fact detail. Writing about how she was retaining water in her muscles, Angella Issajenko observed: "My skin is getting so tight it's hard to push the needle in, also to take it out."

The members of his tightly knit group belonged to what Jamie Astaphan called "the brotherhood of the needle." But now, thanks to the testimony Francis was about to give, the whole country would belong to that fraternity.

As he walked into the Dubin Commission hearing room, Francis tried not to look at the reporters recording his long, loping strides. He also ignored them after he took his seat, got sworn in, and began to tell his life story. His early days as an Olympian. His first meetings with Ben and Eddie, when a meal of French fries seemed like gourmet dining. Their early road-trips through the Great White

North. If he didn't quite come off warm and fuzzy with his deadpan delivery, at least he was seen as something other than his notorious nickname, Charlie the Chemist.

The next day, however, was different. He had to admit to an audience watching on live television that Ben Johnson was, in fact, a steroid user. Johnson had started as far back as 1981, Francis admitted. And, yes, Ben knew that they were banned. Not only did he take them before Seoul, he also took them before his star turn in Rome.

"What informants Joe Valachi did to the mob and Daniel Ellsberg did to the Vietnam War, Charlie Francis yesterday did to sport," David Steen of *The Toronto Star* wrote about the testimony. Another *Star* writer made the same point much less kindly: "Francis' smug recital of wrongdoing was the last word in arrogance. What he laid bare was how thoroughly the rot has set in."

And Francis kept laying it bare over six more days. He revealed that he had been operating with the tacit approval of his country's official body, the Canadian Track & Field Association. And he went on about all the dirty tricks he had seen over the years. There were the athletes who injected themselves with the blood of others to boost their oxygen; the Canadian who said that his British wife, a 100-meter Olympic finalist, was on a 35-milligram-a-day steroid regimen; and the shot-putter who early in Francis's coaching days asked when Francis was going to tell his athletes the "facts of life" and put his sprinters on steroids. "There are people standing up there attempting to claim that they did it clean, they did it by working hard," he said. "And it just isn't true at the highest level," he said.

Those implicated by his testimony were incensed. A rival track coach seethed, "All his life Charlie was a dirty [drug-using] guy as a world-class athlete and as a coach. Now he wants to take everyone else down with him."

By his eighth day before the commission, Francis was weary from all the talk about needles and pills. He had told everything he knew about drugs in sports. In exchange, he didn't want forgiveness. All he wanted was for his critics to concede that he was the best in the world at what he did—no matter how loathsome it might be. Because once they gave him that one piece of cynical praise, they would have to concede that he would never have let a sprinter take a steroid that would have caused a failed drug test in an Olympic final.

It was a corrupt kind of logic. But it was logic, nonetheless.

3

MULES, THREESOMES, AND MOM

March 13, 1989 - May 9, 1989

The federal prison camp in Boron, California, was spread out over hundreds of government-owned acres in the Mojave Desert. The bleached landscape, slithering rattlesnakes, and Gila monsters made it feel like a vacation spot for the damned.

Since William Dillon had recorded conversations with Dan Duchaine on behalf of federal investigators, Duchaine had been on a slow, steady road to junkie oblivion. The once carefree adventurer was gone. This Duchaine spent his days holed up in his apartment, narrowing his circle of friends and partying hardly at all. Wondering who might come for him and when, he started collecting issues of *Soldier of Fortune* and ordered bomb-making manuals. Gun silencers were stored in the upstairs closet. A box of hand grenades lay on his office floor.

There was always a side of him, the actor side, that made it seem like he was just playing at being a drug dealer. It was the side that still had a chance to do what he had originally set out to do in California: direct local theater, try auditioning for small roles, maybe work in a stereo store to pay the rent. It was the side that was sweet and soft-spoken, that never cursed and loved to quote from Jack London's *White Fang*: "One cannot violate the promptings of one's nature without having that nature recoil upon itself." But it was deeply hidden now, very nearly imperceptible. Abandonment had always played a role in Duchaine's life. Being put up for adoption at birth; having his adoptive parents die; loving women who never loved him quite as much. Those were the pillars of his psyche. And the Nubain addiction magnified everything ten-fold so that abandonment went from being an influence to an inevitability. Whatever he did, he was sure he would end up alone. So why not go wild? Why not take more risks? Why not live balls-to-the-wall, even as the feds were closing in?

In early May 1987, when Dillon's help led the feds to bust Duchaine on steroid distribution charges, Duchaine turned to Mike Zumpano, one of the few who remembered, and missed, the Dan of old. He rescued Duchaine once, giving him a job to get him out of Venice. He also put up the $25,000 bail.

"Dan, at what point does a little red light go off in your head telling you that you've gone over the line?" Zumpano wanted to know as they drove back from the federal detention center. Duchaine's answer signaled the yawning distance between them. "I may be going to prison. But you're the one already in prison, with your little life, your little wife."

A few weeks later, Duchaine was arrested again for continuing to deal steroids, causing his bail to jump to $2.5 million. This time he called Zumpano from his detention cell, drugged-out and panicked. "I can't take it in here," he cried. "You have to help me." He pleaded for Zumpano put up his vitamin company as collateral. But there were limits to their friendship. Zumpano told Duchaine no.

Ultimately, Duchaine convinced his aunt Loraine to pledge her house for his bail, and he moved from northern California back to Venice. The feds approached him there about cutting a deal and wearing a wire on his friends. But he would be damned if he was going to go that route after all he had been through. Instead, Duchaine went in the opposite direction. He talked his way into the UCLA Biomedical Library and started reading for hours a day, leafing through old textbooks, veterinary journals, and reports on drugs that were stalling the effects of AIDS. There were few places his curiosity didn't lead him, and few people as well equipped to go there. He became fascinated by whey—a natural protein from cow's milk that was rich in amino acids and contained little fat, making it a highly effective natural supplement for bodybuilders—and started selling it out of his apartment. The cops who were shadowing him became convinced that the large amounts of white powder they saw leaving his place was cocaine, until they stopped a few buyers and realized what was in the bags.

Duchaine was clearly on to something: In later years, whey would become a staple at health food stores. But some of his other discoveries had a cruder edge, and he found a willing audience in a tightly knit group of women bodybuilders.

Women's bodybuilding didn't coalesce as a sport until 1978, when the first-ever women's championship was held in Los Angeles. Its winner was Lisa Lyon, whose sculpted, sinewy look caused a stir among fashion photographers. When Robert Mapplethorpe photographed her nude, with her arms outstretched in a flexing pose and a long willowy sheet draped over her face, the photograph helped Lyon become a female archetype for a new generation. The next year saw the debut of the Ms. Olympia contest, whose winner, Rachel McLish, had cat eyes, high cheekbones, and an ample enough bosom to make her a staple of muscle magazines. Her successor, Corey Everson, reigned from 1984 to 1989 with a look that had slightly more muscular definition yet was still seductive.

As the size of the purses grew, so did the size of the women seeking them. They weren't showing off their figures anymore. They were showing off physiques. Duchaine loved the change. He loved the way these women were more forceful about themselves, more self-aware. They were messing with the status quo. Yet they could also be remarkably docile, especially when it came to taking his advice. Sandra Blackie, a fledgling bodybuilder, recalls getting pills that she knew nothing about, but which Duchaine had promised would help her before a competition. A day after she had swallowed them, she was at the checkout counter of Vaughn's grocery in Venice when she felt dizzy and almost passed out. She returned to his apartment and demanded to know what he'd given her. "It's Glucophage," he said, shrugging his shoulders. He had been reading up on the fact that insulin promotes muscle growth, and decided to experiment with the prescription drug used to treat type 2 diabetes. "Take half as much next time," he said. Blackie walked out stunned at how cavalier he could be, but no less in his thrall.

To Duchaine, Gold's was a supermarket of dysfunctional young women who looked up to him and considered him the stable one. And in the world that he had helped to create—that world of make-believe where people never got married or held day jobs and worked out slavishly so they could carry an ideal of perfection through an imperfect world—perhaps he was. At least he had fallen into some semblance of a stable home life. The woman who had caused the breakup of his first marriage was out, replaced by two others who were living with him. The first was a 21-year-old Air Force officer whom he had met in Gold's; the other was a slightly younger research assistant. After Duchaine married the Air Force officer, Ann Miller, on September 9, 1988, he wrote to his sister, "The girls know each other, accept each other, and actually have become close friends."

Watching television in the 1980s, one would have little idea that people like this even existed. The top-rated drama, *thirtysomething*, was about artsy suburbanites who spent each week wallowing in their self-involvement. For laughs, the choices on the dial ranged from the senior citizen humor of *The Golden Girls* to coming-of-age shows like *Family Ties* and *The Wonder Years*. Unless you counted Hulk Hogan, the cartoonish face of the World Wrestling Federation, there wasn't very much brawn on television.

In fact, America's concept of body image was moving in the opposite direction. In September 1988, Oprah Winfrey created a national sensation by announcing that she was going on a diet with a high-protein, vitamin-packed shake. As more doctors weighed in, the public learned about VLCDs, or very-low-calorie diets, which attacked a growing problem with obesity by supplying as few as 400 calories a day. The diet turned into a national phenomenon. The product's manufacturer reported getting a million calls on its toll-free line and to vendors after Oprah announced she shed 67 pounds on a November 15 show entitled "Diet Dreams Come True." The ratings were the highest in her show's history. *Newsweek* declared: "Oprah: Profile in Curvage."

Four days after that episode aired, in a strange pop culture convergence, *The New York Times* profiled Duchaine on its front page as part of an Olympics-inspired series on steroids in sports. *The Times* scratched the surface of his background, glossing over the creation of the *Underground Steroid Handbook*. But it gave him a chance to cheerlead for steroids in much the same way Oprah was cheerleading for low-calorie shakes. He told the paper that the body builders he studied "who used steroids in conservative amounts appeared to be healthy, with a general feeling of well-being." In other words, he and his friends were living proof that steroids were good for you! Maybe even healthier than Oprah's diet!

He went even further in a column he had begun writing for a new paper to circulate around Venice called *Modern Bodybuilding*. Started by an ex-student from USC, it featured pictures from bodybuilding shows and interviews with muscleheads who were thrilled to find someone so interested in their life stories. Initially, its publisher, Jason Mathas, was wary of Duchaine. A woman he had interviewed at Gold's told him to watch out because "the guy's a freak." Duchaine had leeringly cornered her as she was coming off the stage of a national bodybuilding contest a few weeks earlier and begged her to come to his hotel room, where another of the contestants was tied up with leather and eagerly awaiting a ménage à trois. It didn't stop Mathas from seeking out the Guru, however.

The "Ask The Guru" column was another unqualified hit in the underground, another sign that there was no one quite like Dan Duchaine. Yes, he was going to jail. He had given up fighting and pleaded guilty. But even that struck him as an experience worth having, another thing to cross off his list of things to do before he died. The question was why he felt that way at 35. Why keep counting down, with his life statistically less than halfway over? Why the gnawing sense of fatalism?

The surprising answer came in a phone two months ago from a place he hadn't thought about in years: the Catholic Church that had placed him with his adoptive parents. "Mr. Duchaine," a caseworker said. "We believe we have located your real sister and she'd like to talk to you."

A call was set up with a Connecticut woman named Sheila Butch, who laid out a story that explained everything and nothing at the same time. His real mother, she said, was one of thirteen and had Sheila while waiting tables, but didn't put her up for adoption; she was left with her grandmother until social services intervened and put her in a foster home. Two years later, in 1952, she said her mother became pregnant with Duchaine during an even more troubled period. Documents that Sheila would subsequently acquire showed that her mother had been admitted to New York's Bellevue psychiatric hospital with a diagnosis stark and scary in its simplicity: "The patient is without personality."

Duchaine was immediately put up for adoption (as was another sister who was born two years later). Finally, in the early 1960s, their birth mother married a salesman and moved to Connecticut, regaining custody of Sheila and insisting for the next two decades that her other two children were dead. She maintained this fiction, Sheila continued, until just a few years ago when their mother finally admitted the truth and a long search led Sheila to Dan. "There's one more thing," she said. "I have polycystic kidney disease and so might you."

Duchaine paused. This was before he went to the medical library to learn that polycystic kidney disease involved many (poly) fluid-filled sacs (cysts) growing in the kidneys, eventually squeezing out normal tissue and causing them to fail. All he could think to say was one thing: "I want to talk to Mom."

When he finally called his biological mother, he knew that he had found his wellspring. He could hear it in the blunt, coarse way she spoke, in her rapid-fire manner of storytelling. What shocked him was the story that she had to tell. "Your father was a spy for the CIA," she began, "and we were being chased by the KGB. That's why we had to put you up for adoption." Later, when he recounted it to friends, all he could do was laugh at the prospect of bringing his newfound family to court.

But now it was time to turn himself in. He pulled up to the guard tower at the prison in Boron, took a long drag of the 100-degree Nevada air, and surrendered his California driver's license. The next time he would be a free man, the world would be a very changed place.

TIJUANA, MEXICO
April 1989

If Juan Macklis thought that he had escaped the same fate as Duchaine, he learned otherwise when he arrived to work at his Laboratorios Milanos one day in April. U.S. Customs officials had been pressuring their cross-border brethren to make an example out of the businessman, and after some hemming, they had finally agreed.

Macklis found scores of Mexican police waiting for him, but he had no intention of letting the Americans turn him into a piñata for their quaint drug policies. At about the same time the U.S. Attorney's Office was indicting him, he was recruiting a new moneyman to help him: Manuel Antonio Noriega, the dictator of Panama.

As a Mexican citizen, Macklis didn't have to worry about the indictment that had landed Duchaine in jail. So long as he stayed outside of the United States, there was little the feds could do to him. (Mexico had a long history of not extraditing its citizens.) In fact, he only had to look at Noriega to see how little an American bill of particulars meant. Two separate indictments had been filed against the Latin American leader for cocaine distribution and money laundering. He could not have cared less.

A year earlier, Macklis and Noriega worked out an arrangement that kept the flow of steroids moving. In exchange for an investment of $800,000, Noriega became a co-owner of Laboratorios Milanos while Macklis remained its front man. Macklis would also spend time in Panama, setting up new labs. Since the deal had been struck, the two reaped about $5 million in profits.

Obviously, with friends like that, Macklis had options beyond staying put in Mexico. And shortly after his captors released him, he quietly disappeared from sight.

WASHINGTON, D.C.
May 9, 1989

"The hearing will come to order, please. The press is ready so I am ready." Cameras clicked as Joseph Biden, the 46-year-old senator from Delaware, gaveled the Senate Judiciary Committee hearing to order.

Biden was a full 40 years younger than another senator on the dais, South Carolina's Strom Thurmond, but he had already lived a full political life. He had come into the Senate at the age of 29, and spent the next 16 years preparing to run for President. His chance came in 1988, when he entered a field that included a little-known Massachusetts governor named Michael Dukakis.

Steroids were a perfect apple-pie issue for Biden to reassert himself after he dropped out of the Presidential race when charges emerged that he had plagiarized a campaign speech. With the Ben Johnson scandal still in the public consciousness, the charismatic two-term Democrat introduced a bill that put steroids squarely in the crosshairs of America's war on drugs. It provided a maximum three-year prison sentence for doctors, gym rats, or anyone else who trafficked in steroids for "non-medical" reasons. Ronald Reagan promptly signed the bill.

Unfortunately, there was one thing the 1988 law didn't do. "Several of my colleagues have asked me why we are continuing to focus on this problem," Biden said as the audience settled down. "And they cite, quite correctly, that cocaine and crack in America has become an epidemic and that it is sweeping rural and urban areas around the country. My answer has been simple and direct...."

The new law didn't attack the source: manufacturers. One solution being advanced by certain doctors was to add steroids to the nation's list of controlled substances, and the idea appealed to Biden. Equating steroids to cocaine, another controlled substance, was a perfect way to force the issue here at home.

Unfortunately, Biden was having a hard time finding anyone to agree that steroids met two key definitions of the controlled substances law: that they were addictive and psychoactive. The Department of Health and Human Services Secretary, Otis Bowen, insisted that his research showed that they were neither. Even the normally friendly American Medical Association was having trouble with where things were headed. An Indiana family doctor named Edward Langston, who represented the AMA on the issue, felt compelled to point out that "anabolic steroids do have a role in the treatment of several conditions, including certain anemias, hereditary angioedema, and breast cancer. Moreover, they can be safely used by patients under medical supervision."

Safely used?

At a prior hearing in his home state of Delaware, Senator Biden had presided over some salty testimony. The track star Diane Williams had earned herself an enduring place in the Congressional Record by testifying "my clitoris, which is a penis equivalent, started to grow to embarrassing proportions." And Pat Croce, then a conditioning coach for the Philadelphia 76ers and the Flyers, testified that in order to monitor whether his players had telltale side effects like shrunken testicles, "I tell them to drop their pants and show me how manly they really are."

"In my view," Senator Biden continued, "we did not focus enough attention on the cocaine problem in the late 1970s and early 1980s, with some disastrous results. And it seems to me that we should not make the mistake on this issue...."

To correct that lapse, he put the focus at this hearing squarely on professional sports, particularly the NFL. Lined up to testify were the commissioner, Pete Rozelle; coaches Chuck Noll of the Pittsburgh Steelers and Marty Schottenheimer of the Kansas City Chiefs; the director of the league's players' union, Gene Upshaw; and several players. Speaking to the audience before him—and the one he hoped would re-elect him the next year—the Delaware Democrat made it clear that he believed the sports world bore a specific burden. "The NFL's words and actions, together with those of successful college and pro athletes and coaches around the country, can demonstrate that taking steroids is dangerous, wrong," he began. "For the matter is, tens of millions of we Americans still look to those people who are the stars on the athletic field as the role models in our schools, in our colleges, and in our lives."

Then Biden paused, so his final thought would have time to settle in. "If they are able to benefit from this use without any penalty, then it seems to me the message is overwhelming to the rest of America that drug abuse in any form is not that big a deal."

Biden had drawn a line in the sand. From that point forward, steroids were going to be controlled substances. The era of prohibition had begun.

Now, the real money could be made.

4

THE RUNNING MAN

June 1989 - July 1990

MANHATTAN BEACH, CALIFORNIA

June 1989

Lyle Alzado parked his Rolls-Royce in front of his beachside home at 3220 The Strand and slung his gym bag over his shoulder. Catching a glimpse of himself in the glass, he had to admit that he still had the build that once made him one of the most feared defensive players in the NFL. Still had *the look*.

Only these days, he was stuffing his sculpted body into leather jumpsuits and mink coats, not football pads. Alzado had just wrapped up a season of *Learning the Ropes*, a syndicated sitcom that was being produced in Vancouver. In it, he played Robert Randall, a single dad who was raising two kids while working as a high school vice principal by day and professional wrestler by night. He hated the mechanics of television—memorizing the lines and being fitted for the costumes. Still, it was an improvement on hustling cameos in B movies like *Ernest Goes to Camp*.

He walked through the front door and into the kitchen, where he dropped his gym bag. It felt like a lifetime since he had been on the front lines of the NFL, and certainly more than four years since he had retired. Somewhere he had packed away a photo of himself at Auburn University, where he had been invited to compete in an event called The Strongest Man in Football. The year was 1980 and Alzado had just spent nine years as the defensive star of the Denver Broncos. The competition was one of those cheaply produced ur-reality shows the networks aired to fill an hour on Saturday afternoon. But it was also oddly consequential. The eight men who gathered at Auburn could have been forgiven if they drank beers all day and ogled coeds. But, believe it or not, they actually cared. They cared who could haul the most weight on a flat bench, or dead lift a quarter ton. And so did the crowd that had gathered. Lyle had had bigger nights in his career. Nine months earlier, on July 14, 1979, he had "fought" Muhammad Ali in a charity boxing match. But, looking back, this night was more fateful. Strength was going showbiz.

He had shown up in a white suit with a white fedora and signed autographs for all the college kids, loving every last bit of the attention. He didn't know a thing about the group that was hosting the event—the National Strength Research Institute. Nor had he spent much time around the man with the red beard who was selling tickets, Tony Fitton. (He only loosely made the connection when Fitton was indicted by Phil Halpern for steroid smuggling four years later.) All he cared about was winning. So when he finished eighth, he was crestfallen. He went back to his buddies in Venice Beach and started taking ever-stronger drugs. God, he was crazy in those days. God, he loved being crazy in those days.

He ran his hand through his thinning hair. Perhaps later in the evening he would put on his longhaired toupee and head to a club in West Hollywood. The girls he bought drinks for wouldn't ask him about all the uncomfortable stuff—at least not the young ones. They wouldn't be old enough to remember how it ended in Denver: with the Broncos telling him to shove his salary demands and dumping him onto the Cleveland Browns for draft picks. Certainly, they wouldn't ask how it felt to languish like a fish out of water in the Midwest. If they asked anything, it was usually about the early '80s, when he had resurrected himself as a swashbuckling pirate on the Los Angeles Raiders. Maybe they would ask for a look at his Super Bowl ring. Yeah, the chicks in Hollywood loved the jewelry.

But really, how long could he get off telling old war stories to young girls, bodybuilders, or B-list producers? Some of his most cherished memories were turning into bits that sounded as canned as his TV lines. Even *he* was getting bored with his own career.

Which is why Alzado couldn't get the visit he had just made to Raiders camp out of his head. He had stopped by to say hello to the team's owner, the legendary Al Davis. As they chatted, Davis got on the subject of the days before Alzado retired in 1985.

"The team's not the same as when you were here," Davis told him.

"Not the same," Alzado repeated.

Then a strange pause settled between the two men. It was the kind of pause that said more than either man was prepared to acknowledge.

Was Davis encouraging him to come back? The thought consumed Alzado. He was 40 years old. Could he pull it off? Or more precisely, could he do it in the current climate?

The Ben Johnson scandal had gotten the attention of the United States Congress and convinced several senators that it contained the seeds of a perfect campaign issue. Delaware's Joe Biden had invited several prominent football players to a hearing in the Capitol, including Steve Courson, the ex-offensive lineman for the Pittsburgh Steelers. Courson testified that a "chemical war" was underway in football. Bill Fralic, an offensive lineman with the Atlanta Falcons, went even further by guessing that three-quarters of the linemen, tight ends, and linebackers were probably on the juice.

No shit, Alzado thought. It was exactly 20 years after he had taken his first pill, and they were just getting the message?

How had it started for him? To get an edge? That was a laugh. As a boy, the last thing he needed was an edge. He was all edge. He had his father, Junk Yard Pat, to thank for that.

Junk Yard Pat. The kids in Cedarhurst, Long Island, had given him the nickname because he had kept their large old house filled with junk: rusted appliances, bikes, and car parts. Later in life, when Alzado found out that his father was keeping another family—a girlfriend and four kids—fixed up in Far Rockaway, he would wonder what their house looked like. Did it feel as loveless? Was it as much of a horror show? Sometimes when he went to sleep, Alzado could still hear the sound of his dad's fists on his mother. What little he knew about philosophy and football—the shortest distance between two points is a straight line—he learned from watching his father break his mother's face over and over.

When it came time to leave home, he received no scholarship offers and filtered through a junior college in Texas before landing at Yankton College, a small-town liberal arts school in the South Dakota city of the same name. And from the start, the 190-pound kid Alzado did everything he could to remake himself. He ate yeast pills that expanded his stomach so he could eat nonstop, and lived in the school's weight room.

By his senior year at Yankton, Alzado had added another hundred pounds, and if it wasn't exactly rock, it was enough to turn heads. Any time the school's football team needed a battering ram, it turned to Alzado. The records followed. In 1970, a Denver assistant coach improbably caught some Yankton game film. The Broncos took him in the fourth round of that year's draft.

Somewhere along the line, though, Alzado forgot where that 190-pound kid ended and the drugs began. After his first marriage fell apart in the mid '70s, he started acting like Junk Yard Pat. There was the night he dragged his second wife Cindy out of a Broncos party and pummeled her in their car. And the time she got so angry, she tried to run him over. He had to hang onto the hood of her Toyota for dear life as they sped across Manhattan Beach. (Well, it seemed funny at the time.)

Stories like that helped Alzado gain a reputation as the wildest man in the NFL. But if all the muscle he had put on was a kind of protection from the memory of being a powerless child in an abusive home, it did him no good when he came face-to-face with his father. One night he was in the old neighborhood, visiting a friend, when he looked in the rearview mirror and saw Pat tailing him. Alzado did a U-turn and stared down his grizzled old man through the windshield. For a moment, they looked at one another like rival outlaws in an old B western. Then Alzado sped away, pulling onto a lawn to get past his father's car. His face was covered with sweat.

Alzado figured he had made it when he got traded to the Raiders. He was finally in his city of dreams—Los Angeles. But he was taking so many drugs to fill the hole inside of him that he didn't have time to dream. Bolasterone. Quinolone. Testosterone. His body was working at such warp speed he was lucky if he got four hours of sleep a night. After he led the Raiders to a Super Bowl in the 1983 season, he made a trip to Atlantic City and decided to look up the old man, who by then had divorced both his wives and was living with a new woman. Alzado was being given an award for his work with children, and told Pat as much. The old man just grunted. When his sister, Janice, asked him how the visit went, he seemed crushed. "Dad asked me for money," he said.

Now, in retirement, Alzado was still trying to fill that hole inside of himself, and still taking steroids to do it. He was on Equipoise, a veterinary drug, and Anavar, a mild anabolic steroid. And he still wasn't happy. Who was he kidding? As soon as he heard Al Davis's voice, and the implicit invitation it contained, he knew he wouldn't be able to resist.

He checked the calendar. It was June 1989.

Lyle Alzado had less than a year to get in shape.

NEW YORK CITY

August 29, 1989

Pete Rozelle looked out the window of his Park Avenue office and cursed his luck. In March, he had announced that, after 29 years, he was going to step down as commissioner of the NFL. But the twenty-eight owners of his league couldn't agree on a successor. Rozelle should have been doing a valedictory lap by now. Attendance in the NFL was at an all-time high and the average cost of a franchise was an astonishing $100 million. But instead, the 63-year-old found himself ushering in the 1989 season on the defensive, forced to defend himself against charges that his league was overrun by drugs.

In July, *Sports Illustrated* had hammered him in a story that was highly critical of his chief drug advisor, Forest Tennant. Rozelle was a Madison Avenue man. He knew how to sell. So he had sold Tennant, the owner of a series of California methadone clinics, as the best man for the job. In turn, Tennant trumpeted the fact that the NFL had the toughest drug-testing policy in sports. Last year alone, the league had suspended 24 players for using coke, or pot, or drinking booze.

But steroids were another matter. When Rozelle was named commissioner in 1969, Dianabol was as common as salt tablets. In the San Diego Chargers locker room, bowls of the pink tablets used to be laid out on a table for anyone to take. Much had changed since then. Rozelle had presided over a merger with the American Football League, ushered in *Monday Night Football,* and turned the NFL into a blue-chip entertainment brand. But one thing hadn't changed. It was still remarkably easy for players to find doctors to legally prescribe them *D-bol.*

In the wake of the Ben Johnson scandal, Rozelle tried to stay one step ahead of what he could see was a gathering storm. In 1987 and 1988, NFL players were tested for steroids but were not punished. Rozelle announced that, starting in 1989, anyone caught using steroids would be suspended for four games. It was essentially a Hail Mary play. The players had already learned to beat the test by going off the juice in the preseason and going back on after they had gotten their one test. Only an idiot could fail.

Rozelle didn't need this. What he needed was for the owners to choose his replacement. This morning, however, an interesting piece of news crossed his desk. Thirteen players had flunked their preseason tests for steroids. Obviously, they were mostly the dregs of the dregs. But the number was just large enough that Rozelle could salvage something from this disaster. He could claim his drug-testing program was working. He called the player's union to say he was going public with the list.

God, he'd be happy when this became someone else's problem.

MCLEAN, VIRGINIA
November 1, 1989

The Associated Press story that arrived in the offices of *USA Today* was a small one, and easily overlooked amid the larger news of a bombing in El Salvador, an announcement that President George Bush would meet with Soviet President Mikhail Gorbachev in the Mediterranean, and a deal in Congress to raise the minimum wage to $4.25.

WASHINGTON, November 1, 1989—Anabolic steroids would be placed in the same category as cocaine, a schedule II controlled substance, under a bill proposed Wednesday by Senator Joseph Biden Jr. (D-Del.), chairman of the Senate's Committee on the Judiciary.

The change in designation would allow for increased penalties and tighter regulations.

Reports of steroid use have increased dramatically since Canadian sprinter Ben Johnson was stripped of a gold medal after testing positive at the 1988 Olympic Games in Seoul.

Under Biden's proposal, the Drug Enforcement Administration would have authority to investigate steroid trafficking; the penalty for trafficking would increase from a maximum of three years in prison to 20; and tight production quotas would be imposed.

Steroids are currently considered "prescription drugs" and are regulated by the Food and Drug Administration.

The bill was suggesting a major change. The FDA, which was currently prosecuting steroid dealers around the country, would be out of the loop. In its place, Biden would put the DEA, an agency that didn't consider steroids a controlled substance and didn't want the added responsibility. It was a recipe for disaster. But not many people were prepared to say it.

As it was, an editor at the paper glanced at the dispatch and sent it on to the sports department. There, it was cut down to 52 words and put in the briefs section for the next day's edition. It ran below a headline about a New York Yankee having sex with a 15-year-old girl and the results of the Virginia Slims tennis tournament.

VENICE BEACH, CALIFORNIA
March 1990

As inmate No. 96972-098, Dan Duchaine had done his time without much fuss. He had his favorite bathrobe and slippers sent to him by his doting Aunt Lorraine, and kept to himself in the dorm-like barracks where he was housed, catching up on his reading and answering letters that came in respectable numbers. He spent his nonworking hours in the weight room, or taking long walks up a hill where he could watch fighter jets taking off from the air base next door. The time went mercifully quickly.

When he was released in March 1990, the 38-year-old Duchaine was re-entering a changed world. The Berlin Wall had fallen and the Solidarity movement in Poland was bringing democracy into the heart of the old Soviet empire. But for The Guru, the real tectonic shift came with respect to the laws regarding steroids. Thanks to the efforts of Senator Joe Biden, who had shepherded the Anabolic Steroid Control Act of 1990 through Congress, steroids were now controlled substances, which meant that anyone caught in possession of them without a prescription faced a year in jail; anyone caught dealing could be hit with up to five years in jail for a first offense. Duchaine still believed in steroids enough to recommend them to bodybuilders. But he wasn't going to risk being caught by the feds for selling them, especially when there were so many other drugs to try.

In prison, Duchaine had developed a close friendship with another member of the old Gold's Gym crowd, a former commodities broker named John Romano who was doing time for wire fraud. Romano was the first of the two to be released, and he moved into an apartment complex near the gym in Venice. Duchaine followed him into freedom a month later, and showed up at Romano's doorstep ready to pick up exactly where he had left off.

Romano was patching his ceiling when Duchaine, slightly graying at the temples but still fit, told him to get off the ladder. "You're not going to want to be up there when you try this." Then he held up a syringe with 1.5 units in it and pushed down the plunger to draw out an air bubble.

"That's Nubain, isn't it?" Romano asked.

In prison, Duchaine talked about the drug the way some people talked about their pets. He talked about the smoothness of the high, the way it relaxed him, and how it was a perfect drug for bodybuilding, since it masked muscle aches while suppressing the appetite. Romano looked at the needle warily. He also remembered what Duchaine had told him about what happened when you ran out: the headaches and sneezing, how you didn't want to get out of bed. Duchaine laid the needle on the table and waited for him to pick it up. Romano twirled it between his thumb and forefinger.

"Don't be such a fuckin' pussy," Duchaine snapped. "Just make a fist, point the pin up toward your body, and slide it in. You'll feel it go in the vein. If you see the syringe fill with blood when you pull back on your plunger, you know you're in."

Five minutes after he followed his advice, Romano felt like throwing up. Five minutes after that, Romano felt as though he could lift the world on his back. It was the beginning of a debilitating three-year addiction that went along with being Dan Duchaine's friend.

OXNARD, CALIFORNIA

July 1990

Walking on his hands in the Venice Beach sand, Lyle Alzado realized he was getting used to his life being upside down. Even before he had left Cindy, he had started seeing a new girlfriend, Kris, seriously enough to move her and her two kids into a 10,000-square-foot mansion in Palos Verdes. It became a famous party spot on the NFL circuit, but also a warm one for family. His sister and mom spent a lot of time there, creating one of the few periods of stability in Alzado's life.

Kris had held off marrying Alzado because she knew his history as a husband. But eventually she relented, only to wish she hadn't. One night during a walk through Redondo Beach, Alzado lost his temper and grabbed her by the hair in full view of his sister, dragging her down the street as she screamed. Soon after, Kris filed for divorce.

As he started putting on new muscle and looking like his old self, Alzado became the toast of Hollywood. The film offers started rolling in and he lent his name to a sports bar in West Hollywood that was packed every night. The comeback had turned into such a three-ring circus that *Sports Illustrated* assigned one of its best young writers to follow him.

Shelley Smith was no novice when it came to steroids. She had been at Seoul and was the only reporter to interview Ben Johnson after he had tested positive. Her colleagues at the magazine warned her that Alzado was lying when he said he was drug free. But that was almost beside the point. Smith grew up in Denver in the 1970s and was such a die-hard Alzado fan that she had even slept in a number 77 jersey.

When he took her to Gold's to watch him work out, she became fascinated with his ability to create buzz around himself. Smith wasn't aware of many people who could pull off what Alzado had, or be so simultaneously self-deprecating about it. "You know, you're crazy," she told him.

He smiled back at her. "You think?"

The article that appeared in the July 2 issue of *Sports Illustrated* tried to balance her personal enthusiasm with the skepticism that still surrounded Alzado's improbable comeback. "There are those among the Raider family and the local media who doubt Alzado's motives," she wrote. "The publicity generated by his comeback—newspaper articles and a national talk-show appearance—cannot be bought."

While filming a new NBC show called the *Cutting Edge with Maria Shriver*, Alzado acted like a soldier who wasn't able to make the transition to peacetime. When asked why he was reporting to Raiders camp to compete for a job with men nearly half his age, he replied that it was "real simple—I miss the violence of the game."

Looking at the veins popping from beneath his skin, Shriver, wife of Arnold Schwarzenegger, had to ask the obvious question.

"You know, a lot of people when they see this piece will see that you're 41 years old, you're coming back, you're working out, your standing here in a gym, you look the way you do, they're gonna say, 'The guy's on steroids.'"

Alzado summoned every bit of incredulity he could. "Oh, that's a joke," he replied. "Just because an athlete is built well, and he works hard and he trains hard, it doesn't necessarily mean he has to be on steroids." Then he looked Shriver dead in the eyes as he said, "I'm clean, I've always been clean, and I'm gonna stay clean."

In fact, he was taking a drug that excited him more than any of the others he had used over the years.

Alzado had dabbled with growth hormone in his Denver days, but back then, it was a risky business. The government used human cadavers to extract the drug, a chain of 191 amino acids secreted from the pituitary gland. Gruesome stuff—and dangerous. Who knew what kind of infectious diseases you could get from a corpse? After recipients (usually children who were being treated for dwarfism) started coming down with a rare and fatal condition called Creutzfeldt-Jakob disease (similar to "mad cow" disease in cattle), the European Community ordered it taken off the market. But now a new pair of genetically engineered versions were making the rounds. The muscle magazines were full of stories raving about it. The April 1990 issue of *Muscle & Fitness* carried the cover line, "At Last! Steroid and Growth Hormone Blowout."

Alzado spent $4,000 for a 16-week supply. He also began taking the injectable testosterone cypionate, which was identical to what the body produced naturally, but with one important benefit: it lasted two to four times longer.

At Raiders camp in Oxnard, as Alzado worked through the drills, hitting the stationary pads, he tried to take things slowly and go easy on his rebuilt body. But even with the growth hormone, Alzado couldn't fight time. On the first morning, he felt a twinge in his calf muscle. He tried to straighten himself and it tightened up some more. Nothing to worry about, he told reporters. He'd just take it easy for a while. The next Saturday, it happened again. The muscle was torn.

For the next few weeks, Alzado stayed in his hotel room overlooking the practice facility, watching old movies. When the team left for an exhibition game in England, he stayed behind to have knee surgery, growing ever more depressed. By the time the team got back, the flu that had been lingering was worse. He had a high fever and chills. He had asked his sister Janice what he should do. She told him he was crazy to try to play. But Alzado didn't listen.

There were two preseason games left for him to prove himself, the next one against the Chicago Bears at Soldier Field. Alzado waited to be put into the game. His chance came in the second half, with the Raiders up by 14 points. He found himself in the right place at the right time in the fourth quarter. Chicago's quarterback, Jim Harbaugh, took three steps back, then floated a pass right into Alzado's hands. He ran it back 15 yards, feeling like a little kid until it was nullified by his own offsides penalty. Later on in the locker room, someone pointed out that it was Alzado's first NFL interception. "Yeah, but not the last," he said, brimming with bravado. Four days later, on August 28, he received the news that he had been cut.

Depressed, Alzado returned home and did what he always did when he needed a shoulder to cry on: He called his second wife Cindy and asked her to come to Los Angeles with their son Justin. The three were walking down Melrose Avenue when he stopped at a yogurt shop to buy them smoothies. Grabbing a table where they could all sit, Alzado asked Cindy, "What the hell am I gonna do now?" She had started to answer when he began coughing. It wasn't a mild cough, either. It was the kind that started in his throat and ended up down by his knees. He got up from the table and staggered outside. The next thing Cindy knew, he was unconscious on the sidewalk with blood streaming out of his nose.

It was beginning.

5

INSIDE JOB

August 1990 - March 1991

VENICE BEACH, CALIFORNIA

August 1990

It didn't take Dan Duchaine long to resume his career as a writer and trainer, with Romano as his newest protégé. Mornings would begin with a wake-up shot of Nubain and a dose of Fastin, a weight-loss pill that was one of his new discoveries. As soon as their eyes popped open, it was off to Gold's, where bodybuilding was going through another periodic shift. Muscle magazines reflected it by putting gargantuan new stars on their covers with lines like "Gladiator Delts," "Killer Calves," and "Blast Furnace Intensity."

These were prolific days for Duchaine as he experimented with drugs such as vanadyl, metformin, Fastin, Nolvadex, HGH, and clenbuterol. On any given day, his Vernon Street apartment might be filled with porn stars, mobsters, bouncers, an AIDS researcher, or even a mortician. It had become a kind of Pasteur Institute for the freak parade.

But one day, a woman walked into the Institute who made

Duchaine forget about all the others. Shelley Harvey wasn't as bombastic as the other women he knew. In fact, she was positively reserved by the standards of the usual crowd. The 27-year-old had grown up in the heart of London, with trips to the theater and all the other prerequisites of a well-attended young girl. Somewhere along the way, though, Harvey had discovered bodybuilding. And having won several small titles, she had flown to Venice to ask The Guru to take her to the next level.

Harvey fell for Duchaine the moment that she laid eyes on him. His jet-black hair was grown down to his back, tied in a long ponytail, and he dressed in tight jeans and a tight-fitting tee. "He looked like a rock star," she would recall years later. But as they got to know one another, he wasn't the figure she imagined. He was quiet and kind, attentive in a way she wasn't used to seeing from men who earned their living in gyms. That first night, they went to dinner and a film in Westwood. They spent all of the next day together, and the day after that, and the day after that. As she got to know him, Harvey was struck by the hardness of his life. She nearly cried when he described the Christmases he had spent alone as a boy—buying his own tree, decorating it without help, and reading quietly beside its light while all the other homes in his Maine town were bustling with family celebrations. He told such stories without the slightest trace of pity, which made Harvey determined to love him even more. Instead of returning home, she stayed with him for good.

Their home life managed to be both ordinary and extraordinary. The two watched television like any other couple, but their chitchat inevitably ended up at who they thought was on the juice. Flicking through the channels, Harvey got a running commentary, from which female pop star Duchaine thought had a chemical secret to which fading action star was getting help from a needle.

Harvey also learned that being with Duchaine meant trying all the drugs that he was experimenting with. And none was more grippingly addictive than GHB, the drug he boasted to friends "helps me have the best sex I've ever had."

Researchers conducting experiments on the human brain in 1960 were the first to synthesize gamma hydroxybutyrate. Since its structure is similar to an amino acid that the body produces naturally to induce sleep, it was initially considered a promising anesthetic. But then a UCLA researcher decided to give large doses of it to cats. What he saw was unforgettable. A video of his experiment shows the cats experiencing spasmodic episodes, their tails standing up at unnatural angles. The researcher concluded that the drug worked by bombarding the brain with hallucinatory images, causing it to overload and enter a deep stage of sleep.

The research caused such a stir in the medical community that drug companies like Sigma decided to end their clinical trials of it. But three decades later, GHB was making a comeback, thanks to an Arizona chemist with an affinity for tear gas and a make-believe doctor who was linked to a clinic that froze heads.

Mark Thierman, a 28-year-old chemist, owned a Tucson-based company called Amino Discounters Limited that sold the most GHB in America. Thierman stumbled onto the drug after reading an obscure Japanese study from the late 1970s that found that it caused users to enter a deep stage of sleep during which growth hormone production increased. Knowing a good sales pitch when he saw one, Thierman began selling GHB as a kind of magic elixir to health food stores and muscle magazines such as *Ironman* under the name Somatomax P.M. After a while, he also started gearing the product to a group of cultists who believed in the strange and sometimes shadowy science of life extension.

Thierman's gateway to the group was a Palm Springs scientist named Larry Wood. Well-built and well-spoken, the 43-year-old Wood believed in better living through chemistry. But he also believed in hedging his bets. If science wasn't currently up to the task of helping him live a hundred more years, he wanted to be around when it was. His belief in living forever led him to a Scottsdale, Arizona, company called the Alcor Life Extension Foundation (which years later would become famous for cryogenically freezing the head of Ted Williams). Its co-owner had just been investigated for having his 83-year-old mother's head cut off in the hope that freezing it would allow him to reattach her to a new body in the future. There was initially some question about whether the ailing woman was actually dead before her head was detached, but a coroner found that she had died first of pneumonia and the case eventually got closed without charges being lodged.

Wood aligned himself with Alcor as a consultant, looking out for new products that could fit its core beliefs. By that spring, thanks to a loose association with Thierman,[1] he was also marketing GHB.[2]

Wood knew Dan Duchaine through his writings and thought it might help business if he gave GHB a try. A few days after Duchaine received a sample, Wood's phone rang: "Jesus, Larry," Dan said. "This stuff is great."

LOS ANGELES
September 22, 1990

Kathy Davis pulled up to Lyle Alzado's restaurant at 826 North La Cienega Boulevard and handed her keys to the parking valet. A few weeks earlier, she had come here with a girlfriend and was shocked when the restaurant's namesake sat down at her table and began talking for two straight hours. Davis, a young model, didn't know much about football. But she was struck by how much attention Alzado lavished on her and welcomed his suggestion that she come back to the restaurant for a real date, just the two of them.

---

1 Wood started buying his GHB from a San Francisco middleman named Stan Antosh, who initially suggested using Duchaine to publicize the drug.
2 At first, he was moving just a few hundred bottles a week. But then the law of unintended consequences intervened, and a government crackdown on another supplement opened a whole new market for GHB. The crackdown involved L-tryptophan, a popular sleep aid. A bad batch had just hit the streets, causing 38 deaths and an emergency FDA ban. Suddenly a lot of people who had grown reliant on L-tryptophan were getting strung out. Wood pitched GHB as an alternative.

She was a bit irked that it took three weeks to arrange, but Alzado explained it away by saying he had to be briefly hospitalized for a silly little injury.

Over dinner that night, and many more in the months to come, Alzado confessed to being at a crossroads. The bit parts in movies were still pouring in and keeping him busy, but it wasn't football. The challenge wasn't the same. Maybe, she suggested, what he needed was to settle down. In the early fall, she took him to her parents' home in Portland and showed him how a small-town family lived. His eyes grew wide. For the first time, he started imagining another kind of life for himself.

Alzado kept certain things from Davis. Kris was one of them. He conveniently left out his third marriage because he didn't want the two women anywhere near one another. His steroid use was another. One day Davis saw a needle in his bathroom of his Manhattan Beach house and asked about it. "Don't worry," he said, dismissing it. "Everyone I know takes them." She accepted the explanation, in part because she saw no negative effects. But that changed after they had been dating a few months. She went to visit him on the set of a movie he was filming, *Neon City*. It was a junky sci-fi flick about survivors of a military experiment that had created a solar disaster and Lyle had secretly upped his dose of the drugs to look good for his role as the ex-con, Bulk.

During a break in filming, a crewmember was helping Davis across a mud puddle when Alzado caught sight of them. Without thinking, he ran toward them like he was back on the football field, except that instead of a quarterback his target was a lowly assistant. Alzado grabbed him by his shirt and threw him against a wall, his face so flushed that he could barely spit out the words, "You ever touch her again.... " After Alzado was pulled away, Davis was hysterical. "Is that what a 'roid rage looks like?" she screamed in his trailer. "Because if it is, I never want to see it, or you, again!"

For the most part, Alzado was able to keep his promise to avoid a repeat. There were no similar flare-ups and he made sure that his used needles were kept out of Davis's sight. On Halloween night, he proposed to her on the pier at Manhattan Beach.

She couldn't say yes fast enough.

For the wedding, Davis arranged an intimate ceremony in a church near her parents' home. It was a very un-Hollywood affair where the groom wore a simple black tuxedo and the bride wore a traditional white dress. Thanks to the divorce with Kris and the child support payments that he was forever late in making to Cindy, the newlyweds didn't have much money. So they spent their honeymoon at a cabin in the hills that her parents had given them for a week as a present. After a post-wedding breakfast, Alzado handed her the keys to their car. "Here, you drive," he said. "I'm feeling kind of tired from last night."

The couple decided to venture out to a movie. Alzado, of course, was instantly recognized, first by a young boy who asked for his autograph, then by another and another. He dutifully signed all of their slips of paper until he saw them looking strangely at what he had given them back. It was then that he noticed his usually purposeful signature was just circles. "Something's wrong, Kathy," he said. "I can't control my hands."

The couple cut their honeymoon short to fly back to Los Angeles. Alzado thought he might be suffering from an inner ear infection because his balance was off during the flight and Davis had to help him walk. As soon as they returned to his home in Manhattan Beach, she started looking through all his drawers, searching for medicines he might have been taking, anything that she could show a doctor. What she found stunned her.

Her husband of less than a week had collected enough drugs to open two pharmacies—one for humans and another for farm animals. He had five types of oral anabolic steroids and 16 types of injectable ones. Some had pictures of horses on the box, suggesting they were veterinary medicines. Others had labels from East

Germany, West Germany, Mexico, France, Italy, and the United States. She dropped everything in a brown bag and took Alzado to a doctor who knew him all too well.

VENICE BEACH, CALIFORNIA
October 1990

Dan Duchaine's first mention of GHB occupied a single paragraph in the October 1990 issue of *Modern Bodybuilding*. Later that month, Larry Wood was moving $10,000 worth of the stuff a week. He might have continued making that kind of money for a while if not for one problem: Like a smoldering fire, it was nearly impossible to control. A two-gram dose of GHB might produce a good night's sleep, but above that, the drug started taking over.

As GHB's unofficial ambassador, Duchaine had already discovered as much. He was giving it to anyone who was interested. It didn't take long for bodybuilders who doubled as bouncers to introduce it into the clubs and give it to their girlfriends, who happily saw it as a great low-calorie alternative to booze. (Another thing that recommended GHB was that users who got pulled over by the cops would pass a Breathalyzer test, provided they hadn't mixed the drug with alcohol.)

By the fall of 1990, the party crowd's embrace of GHB was starting to yield some frightening results. Clubgoers were taking ever-larger doses, mixing it with other party drugs. The effects were being seen in hospitals from California to Georgia, where healthy people were being wheeled in frothing at the mouth while their bodies convulsed. In November 1990, California's health director leapt into action by ordering a statewide ban on GHB sales. Two weeks later, the feds got in on the act, launching an investigation that Thierman knew would eventually reach him.

On a brisk fall evening, Wood pulled up to Thierman's lab in a rented Ryder truck and loaded nearly a half-ton's worth of pure GHB, stored in canisters, into the back. Then he drove the booty off to another warehouse in Phoenix, beating the feds' arrival to Tucson by a few days. When the FDA agents finally arrived, they didn't know about the missing cache. But they found enough—including scales, cash, and documents—to convince them that Thierman was worth keeping an eye on. Undaunted, the chemist simply moved his lab to another location on the other side of town, mopping the floors of the one he'd abandoned with tear gas to spite the feds in case they returned.

Wood, meanwhile, continued to sell the magic liquid openly. And on December 13, it was Wood's turn to be targeted. Federal agents who had discovered records linking him to Thierman carted off guns that were locked in Wood's floor safe, $25,000 in cash, and boxes of pills that he had in his garage. After spending a night in the local jail, he was badly shaken. But not so shaken as to hang up on an Ohio man who had called looking for a score.

"Look pal," Wood said, "I've just been raided and spent the night in jail. This isn't a good time. Call me back." In mid-February, Wood faxed him back to say he was ready to talk. "There's not a lot of stuff out there right now," he said when the two made contact on February 19, "but there's a guy I know who might be able to help. I'll have him call you."

VENICE BEACH, CALIFORNIA
March 14, 1991

After a workout and breakfast, Dan Duchaine showered, kissed Shelley goodbye and jumped on his scooter to head to a storage locker that he kept on South Fourth Street. Roughly the size of a large bedroom, he had outfitted it with a stereo system, armchair, and enough magazines to fill three doctors' offices. Classical music was playing on the stereo when he took ten 50-gram bottles and another ten 100-gram bottles of GHB, along with 50 tablets of clenbuterol, and placed them in a small cardboard box. Then he wrapped it in brown shipping paper and addressed it to the Ohio man whom he had called at Wood's suggestion, Bill Sands.

CENTURY CITY, CALIFORNIA

March 1991

Robert Huizenga had received his medical degree from Harvard, but he did his steroid residency in the school of Lyle Alzado. As the team doctor for the Raiders, he often traveled to road games. One day during the 1983 season, he walked past Alzado's hotel room and saw syringes on his discarded food tray. When he asked the star about them, Alzado was nonplussed. "Rob, you have to understand," he said. "My brother is less than 200 pounds. I can't play at that size."

Alzado regarded Huizenga as someone who could do him no good, someone who would be concerned about steroid abuse. Huizenga, in turn, saw Alzado as a ticking time bomb. A good HDL cholesterol level would be between 40-50. In 1983, Alzado's was in the single digits, putting him at huge risk for a coronary episode. When Huizenga saw the defensive end go down in his final game in 1985, he rushed onto the field, praying that it was something treatable, like a ruptured Achilles tendon, and not a fatal heart attack.

During Alzado's attempted comeback, the old foes were reunited. "You know, it's not like 1985," Huizenga had told him. "The NFL is testing for lots of new things now. Masking agents. Diuretics. You can't pull your old tricks." Alzado flashed his old, confident grin and replied: "Don't worry about me, doc. I can take care of myself." Alzado clearly had the V-shaped look, the acne, and the mood swings that suggested he was on the stuff. And though Huizenga didn't have the kind of proof that would allow him to take action with the team, he had no doubt that Alzado could beat a drug test. And when he was given his mandatory preseason NFL drug test, he passed it with flying colors.

When the comeback bid failed, Huizenga didn't expect to hear from Alzado again. So he was surprised when he came to see him after the yogurt shop incident, wanting to know why he couldn't shake his nasty cough. X-rays didn't provide the answers, but Huizenga did get one mystery solved. How had Alzado beaten the new drug tests? With nothing left to hide, Alzado was matter-of-fact. He had taken oral steroids, he explained, which cleared the body quickly, until just before training camp. Then he switched to human growth hormone, for which there was no test.

Now, six months later, Alzado was back in Huizenga's medical office in Beverly Hills, describing why he had had to cut his honeymoon short. Davis dumped the brown bag on his desk and asked if the drugs could have had something to do with it. Huizenga tried to hide his astonishment at what was inside. "Where'd you get all this stuff?" he asked. Alzado told him that most of it came from a pair of East German trainers he had used during his comeback.

Huizenga made an appointment for Alzado to get an MRI at the UCLA Medical Center. And late in the afternoon, he read the results with horror. It looked like there were mothballs floating in the fluid in his brain. It was the kind of thing he had seen before in patients with AIDS, but never in a football player. Rushing to Alzado's room, Huizenga peppered his patient with questions. Had he ever had homosexual sex, visited prostitutes, or used intravenous drugs? Lyle looked confused and afraid in his hospital whites with his toupee off. "No, doc," he answered each time.

"Well, Lyle, there's something very strange going on."

Given Alzado's answers, Huizenga discounted HIV. But a biopsy of his brain showed that he had cancer. Alzado had wanted to start a new life with Davis. Yet if the most sobering predictions were correct, they would be lucky to have a year together.

Alzado immediately started undergoing radiation therapy and wearing a black eye patch to stop the dizzy spells that kept him from sitting upright. The bald and patched look made a sad mockery of the pirate image that Alzado had cultivated on the Raiders.

His illness also put a strain on their finances. The couple decided to give up their fancy apartment for a single bedroom in Beverlywood and were living among boxes when, at 7:00 on the morning of April 16, a knock came on the door. Alzado wasn't sleeping well and the intrusion put him into a rage. He flung open the apartment's door to find a deputy marshal with a subpoena for him to appear at a civil court hearing on a business deal that had gone bad. Alzado cursed at the marshal and then, feeling dizzy, stumbled toward her. Mistaking his lurch as an act of aggression, the 110-pound deputy emptied a can of Mace in his face.

Until that moment, Alzado had jealously guarded his privacy. He was even keeping his family at arm's length. But now, in this senseless and patently ridiculous moment, that was about to change.

The marshal came back with sheriff's deputies and, after briefly stopping at a hospital to treat him for his Mace burns, dragged Alzado down to the Marina Del Rey stationhouse. With no interest in protecting him, the cops put out word that a former football great had been arrested.

A story in the April 17 edition of the *Los Angeles Times* treated the incident almost humorously. "Lyle Alzado, an imposing former Raiders defensive lineman, found himself overmatched Tuesday in an early morning encounter with a 110-pound female deputy marshal armed with a can of chemical Mace and some law enforcement friends, according to authorities."

For Alzado, it was the ultimate insult. Even in his weakened state, he couldn't handle being humiliated like that. So on April 19, he allowed his attorney to draft a release that acknowledged the truth. "Mr. Alzado was incapable of committing any of the alleged acts purported to have occurred," it said. Huizenga was on hand to supply the reason: brain cancer. His patient, he said, is "quite unsteady when he walks."

With the press hovering, Alzado hid in his apartment. The illness was getting worse and he was starting to have regular seizures. He had just finished throwing up in the bathroom when he caught a glimpse of himself in the mirror. At first, he didn't recognize the man who was staring back. Then it hit him. The person looking back at him wasn't a stranger. It was the scrawny kid who had left Long Island behind some 24 years earlier.

It took cancer to do it, but Lyle Alzado was finally being reunited with his old self.

6

BLOW OUT

May 17, 1991 - October 31, 1991

Shelley Harvey was in the kitchen of the apartment she shared with Dan Duchaine, fixing an egg-white omelet, when a loud boom made her drop the frying pan and singe her forefinger. Still shaking it, she ran into the living room to see her boyfriend getting pinned to the floor by U.S. marshals. "I'm really sorry, Shelley," he said as the marshals started ransacking the place, but not finding anything except a hollowed-out book filled with cash.

Bill Sands was, in fact, an undercover FDA agent and the package he had received from Duchaine gave the feds all the evidence they needed to obtain a search warrant to search his apartment. They came in with guns drawn and carted him away. "What the hell happened?" Romano asked when Duchaine called him from jail. It wasn't a completely selfless question. Romano had testosterone stored under a floorboard and was scared they were going to nab him, too.

"They think they can fuck with me," Duchaine answered, "but I ain't no pussy." At worst, he figured he was facing a misdemeanor rap for mislabeling, a nuisance charge. He was more worried about Harvey finding out what he'd been doing; he had kept that part of his life separate from her. But he underestimated the forces aligning against him.

On June 6, an indictment was unsealed that accused him and Wood of conspiracy to defraud the federal government. Defraud the government? With one conviction to his name already, the new charge could send him away for years.

SAN PEDRO, CALIFORNIA
June 1991

Sports Illustrated writer Shelley Smith was sitting at her home in San Pedro, trying to line up her next article, when one of her editors called from New York with a tip: The magazine had heard that Lyle Alzado was dying and might be ready to come clean about his long-rumored steroid use.

A year earlier, Smith had greeted Alzado's comeback with the same enthusiasm she had felt during his playing days in Denver. But since it sputtered out, she had moved on in her career, writing about horseracing, surfing, and college basketball. A story about steroids just wasn't on her radar.

Smith called Alzado's camp and suggested that her magazine would be willing to do a first-person piece with him, if indeed he had something he wanted to get off his chest. A few back-and-forths later, an interview was arranged at his agent's home, a cream-colored residence in Beverly Hills once owned by Charlie Chaplin.

When she pulled up in her Honda, Smith took a deep breath and gathered herself together before getting out. Between the millionaire superstars, the crestfallen losers, and the emotional hucksters that a journalist comes across, you couldn't afford to lose yourself in your work too much. Smith had learned how to protect herself from that. But she had never stuck a tape recorder in front of a dying man before.

Smith rang the bell and was led in to find Alzado waiting for her on the couch. His positioning wasn't accidental. Alzado could hardly walk and he didn't want to frighten her by teetering unsteadily on his feet. As it was, Smith had to catch herself so she wouldn't seem shocked by his transformation. The last time they had met, Alzado was a mountain of a man. Now, the same clothes he had worn then were hanging off his frame like sacks. His cheeks were sunken and the eyes that used to be so fiery had another look in them: fear. He gave her as hearty a handshake as he could manage.

As they sat down, Smith stared at a flowing black-and-red scarf that Alzado had wrapped around his head. A few months earlier, he had been in a mall when he noticed a bald-headed boy of maybe 12 whom he instantly took for a fellow chemotherapy patient. He handed the boy his Raiders cap, and they talked for a while. Then, when he got home, he rooted through his closet to find something to replace it. What he came across was the silk scarf that Davis had bought in a London thrift store years before. Smith thought it looked curiously stylish. Even now, Alzado was making a statement.

After some small talk ("What do you think of my hair now?" he quipped), she placed a tape recorder before him. "Are you sure you want to do this?" she asked. He said he was sure.

Smith tried not to dwell on the sad fact that Alzado's cancer was the last bit of celebrity currency he had left. Or that, in his final months, he had come to the conclusion that he wanted to be remembered for disavowing what he had once stood for in life. Those were difficult and powerful realizations to face. But maybe the morphine was easing his emotional pain, as well.

Smith pressed the record button on her machine, and slid it in front of Alzado. He began speaking slowly and steadily, making the most shocking steroid confessions that she or any other sportswriter had ever heard.

When they were finished, Smith felt drained and profoundly sad. She thanked Alzado and assured him that she would do the best she could to bring not just his words, but his voice to her magazine's more than 20 million readers. It was a huge task and one she took seriously.

That night at home, Smith began transcribing her tape. When she was done, she didn't look at that transcript. Instead, she glanced out her office window at the Pacific Ocean and closed her eyes, forcing herself to hear Alzado's voice in her head. She wanted his most important words to come to her naturally.

When the magazine hit the stands on June 8, his story led with what had echoed in her head at that moment:

"I lied. I lied to you. I lied to my family. I lied to a lot of people for a lot of years when I said I didn't use steroids."

DETROIT
June 20, 1991

In the three years since Dennis Degan had first helped put Dan Duchaine behind bars, business had been good for the FDA agent. A diagram sat on his desk that showed his office in the center of a grid, orbited by nearly 30 other law-enforcement agencies to which he had fed raw intelligence. He had single-handedly turned his Detroit office into a case factory and there was no end in sight.

He and a staff of 10 aides worked around the clock to create a database of dealers that rivaled anything the CIA was compiling on the Middle East. With a specially requisitioned computer that cost $100,000, Degan was able to catalog every name he had ever come across in a steroid probe. If an address book was seized in a raid, he would have his staff input all the names and cross-check them against other documents they had collected. The walls of his office were lined with two-tier file cabinets crammed full of thick black binders containing 750,000 pages—350 linear feet—of investigative material. It ranged from grand jury testimony to search warrant applications to notes from informants.

Nothing in the history of steroid prosecutions approached what Degan had done because there was no other history; he was making it as he went along. The case he was most proud of involved a 28-year-old Iranian who was the world's leading exporter of counterfeit drugs. A U.S. Attorney working with Degan had convinced several major drug companies to put up $30 million as bait to catch the dealer in a sting at London's posh Dorchester Hotel. It was the largest such operation that the FDA had ever undertaken and a major success.

The bushy-bearded agent had also become a staple of the commission circuit. He had testified before Congress, as well as before Canada's famed Dubin Commission.[1] Yet despite all of this, Degan found himself fighting to keep his job. A few months earlier, Congress enacted the bill that had been introduced by Senator Joe Biden, officially adding steroids to the nation's controlled substances list. That should have been good news for someone like Degan, who was uniquely positioned to help. But the exact opposite was turning out to be true. The bill created a raging debate in the upper reaches of the FDA at precisely the time a new commissioner was taking over its reins.

In a series of hearings, Congress was accusing the FDA of losing its way, neglecting bread-and-butter issues like drug regulation. So the Bush Administration turned to an aggressive lawyer/doctor named David Kessler to shake things up. Kessler, a pediatrician by training, wasted no time talking tough. "We have a lot to do here," he told Congress during his first appearance on March 7. "It will take my entire tenure, and it will go beyond one commissioner."

---

1 Degan also communicated with Charlie Francis, who kept insisting that Ben Johnson had been framed and was trying to interest him in a probe of Carl Lewis, but there was no evidence against Lewis and Degan declined.

His agenda, however, seemed to not include steroids. It wasn't that he didn't recognize the danger of abuse; it was that the Drug Enforcement Administration, with its statutory duty to police controlled substances, seemed better suited to the task. Kessler didn't want his people trying to compete with real cops by carrying around guns and busting down doors.

Degan felt that was a dangerous miscalculation. The DEA was worried about cocaine and heroine dealers; its people would put steroids on the bottom of its priority list. He had finally gotten U.S. Attorneys from around the country to get serious about the steroid issue. This wasn't the time to change strategy.

In fact, his bosses only had to look at that morning's *USA Today* to see what kind of a roll he was on. It was right there on the front page, under the headline, "Hulk: Bulk from a Bottle?" The accompanying story was about a rogue doctor who was going on trial in Pennsylvania for supplying steroids to members of the World Wrestling Federation. Degan had personally helped to make the case, and it was a first step in exposing the role of steroids in the entertainment industry. (Another doctor, Walter Jekot, would soon plead guilty to an indictment of conspiracy to receive and distribute steroids. Jekot boasted a patient list of athletes and celebrities, which, according to court records, included *Baywatch* star David Hasselhoff.)

Degan threw some clothes into a suitcase and got ready to head to Harrisburg. Damn what they said in Washington, he thought. *This* is how you fight a drug war.

HARRISBURG, PENNSYLVANIA
June 25, 1991

George Zahorian lived the life of a prominent doctor in Harrisburg. But his slicked-back hair and colorful tuxedos suggested a man who had a taste for a more flamboyant lifestyle than western Pennsylvania could provide. Fortunately, he had found an outlet in an arcane state law that treated professional wrestling as a real sport.

The original artisans of wrestling—the stars that Zahorian grew up watching near New York City in the 1950s—took enormous pride in their ability to fool the public. Under strict rules set down by the old-time promoters, wrestling's heroes and villains, otherwise known as babyfaces and heels, couldn't be seen together when they were away from the ring. In many cases, wrestlers wouldn't even let their families in on the secret. But a cleft-chinned, third-generation promoter named Vincent McMahon changed those rules. After buying the World Wide Wrestling Federation from his father in 1983, he had started phasing out the pulp heroes in favor of a new breed of showman typified by Terry Bollea, a Tampa guitarist with a beach bum tan who had found a second life as a wrestler.

If Arnold Schwarzenegger seemed to be chiseled from stone, Bollea, who wrestled under the name Hulk Hogan, looked as if he had been drawn in an animation studio. His 22-inch arms were the stuff of cartoons, and he didn't act so much as mug, bug-eyed, for the camera. Hogan wasn't the most artful wrestler to set foot in the squared circle, but after learning how to take pratfalls in VFW halls from Memphis to Minneapolis, he was shrewd. Like McMahon, he hated the old-school types who treated wrestling as an earnest art form. He wanted it to rock and roll.

Hogan got his chance when Sylvester Stallone caught a glimpse of him wrestling on TV and offered him the part of a seven-foot wrestling champ called Thunderlips in 1982's *Rocky III*. As soon as the film debuted, fans started flocking to see the larger-than-life Hogan wrestle in person. (The movie's producers had billed him as being seven inches taller than his actual six-foot-five size, literally heightening his allure.) Soon, McMahon was pairing his star with a quirky new pop star named Cyndi Lauper in a series of kitschy clips that culminated with a match televised on MTV, *The Brawl to Settle It All.*

The crossover helped the WWF become a mainstream attraction, and helped McMahon's other stars—Randy "Macho Man" Savage, Rowdy Roddy Piper, the indefatigable Iron Sheik—sell lunch boxes to kids, tickets to their parents, and ratings to cable and network television executives. By the late '80s, the little company that McMahon ran from Stamford, Connecticut, was a juggernaut. He'd even sunk $20 million into a big-budget action vehicle for Hogan, *No Holds Barred.*

Since the WWF filmed its weekly show at a studio in Allentown, Zahorian jumped at the chance to work in the part-time employ of the Pennsylvania Athletic Commission, which required that a doctor be stationed ringside at all wrestling matches. Once a month, he trotted out to the tapings at the old fairgrounds, dressed to the nines in the hope that the camera might catch him bandaging a wrestler who had been hurled into a turnbuckle, or mopping blood from someone's brow.

Had that been the extent of his involvement, he would have been little more than an eccentric country doctor. But Zahorian had become a bargaining chip in someone else's game. A strength coach from the University of Virginia named Bill Dunn had been buying steroids from Zahorian for much of the 1980s, and was peddling that information for a deal on his drug charge. He tried offering the doctor up in late 1987, but the cops who arrested him in Chesapeake, Virginia, didn't much care. It wasn't until Dunn was awaiting sentencing in early 1989 that Zahorian suddenly had value.

At the time, Degan had been working with a Justice Department official who was interested in pursuing doctors. When they heard that a washed-up strength coach was ready to name a well-connected Pennsylvania doctor, they decided that they had found a perfect "target of opportunity."

In October 1989, Degan taped a small recorder to Dunn's back and sent him into Zahorian's office with $650 and a shopping list of steroids to buy. "Man, you look good," Zahorian said when he saw his old patient.

"Tryin' to stay healthy," Dunn replied.

"So, what do you think you'll need?" Zahorian asked.

Dunn unfurled a list of drugs and watched Zahorian fill it. "I'm giving you better prices than the wrestlers," the doctor said. "But I know you, okay? I'll make it worth your while."

Sitting in a van outside, listening to the exchange, Degan wondered what he meant. *The wrestlers?* Who were they?

He found out six months later, when they sent Dunn back to make an even bigger buy. The snitch found Zahorian more nervous than he had been six months earlier. He had heard through sources in the WWF that the feds were nosing around his affairs, and he was rattled. "I'm not carrying as much as I used to," he said. "I don't see wrestlers anymore. I don't see anybody. I don't need it. I don't need the aggravation. I mean, they're watching the wrestlers very close. Very close." Zahorian then proceeded to give Dunn more drugs than a small army could use: 60 Vicodins, 1,128 Halcions, 952 Xanax tablets, 48 Limbitrols, four vials of testosterone, and 85 Darvocets. Dunn handed him a gym bag with $25,000 in cash.

As soon as the buy was made, Degan leapt from his van with a search warrant in hand. The doctor went pale when he saw Degan at his door, accompanied by an FBI agent. He begged for time to call his lawyer and stepped back into his waiting room. But with the door half open, Degan could see that Zahorian wasn't calling anyone; he was ripping up documents.

Now, 13 months later, the doctor was going to have to convince a jury why he had done that, and why Rowdy Roddy Piper's name was among those on the FedEx receipts he had tried to shred. Degan had tightened the noose by subpoenaing all of Zahorian's other FedEx records, which contained evidence of dozens more deliveries to wrestling stars. Many were shipped to hotels and cities where the company toured, but a dozen more made their way to the Stamford, Connecticut, building from which McMahon ran his company.

When Degan arrived in Harrisburg, the U.S. district court building was as much of a circus as one of McMahon's shows. Media were camped out, hoping to catch sight of Hogan coming in. As it happened, a feverish round of last-minute negotiations allowed him to escape being subpoenaed, and only Piper was left to testify. Still, Degan took comfort in seeing the coverage the case was getting. When he had started, no one had thought steroids were important. Now, their connection to the most popular show on cable television was causing media apoplexy.

As the trial got underway, Degan waited in the U.S. Attorney's Office, anticipating being called as a witness. But that turned out not to be necessary. The case was so airtight that the prosecutors trying the case decided they didn't need him. Degan, therefore, never heard Zahorian testify that he was really a saint of sorts.

"I knew these individuals," Zahorian told the jury. "I treated these individuals. I had carried out physicals and histories on them. They were taking minimal amounts of medication that was given to them in minimal doses. I knew it wasn't going to harm them. Over the 10 years that I knew most of the individuals, not one was sick, not one developed anything that stopped them from wrestling."

It was just as well. By that point, Degan had heard enough self-justifications. He didn't need to hear one more. More importantly, he had work to do back in Detroit that necessitated him catching the next flight home. Had he stuck around, though, he wouldn't have lost much time.

The jury got the case at 1:30 p.m. on June 25. It only took them three hours to decide that Zahorian was guilty of pumping up Hulk Hogan and the other wrestling stars.

MISHAWAKA, INDIANA
July 3, 1991

In a summer of boring sequels, Arnold Schwarzenegger was about to deliver a blockbuster. He was promoting it everywhere: at a plant that was producing a monstrous new vehicle called a Hummer; on the cover of *Muscle & Fitness* magazine; while judging an Arnold look-alike contest; while presiding over the Hollywood premiere; and while telling an interviewer on CBS that he had no interest in running for governor of California in 1994. "Why would I?" he asked, deferring to his duties on the President's council on physical fitness. "The most important thing for me is right now to make America healthy."

As Dave Kehr noted in the *Chicago Tribune*, Hollywood was churning out "the kind of female-centered melodrama that has been revived by Julia Roberts." But Schwarzenegger's new movie, *Terminator 2*, was about to fly in the face of that trend. Though clearly a star vehicle for Arnold, the $102 million epic was built around the character played by Linda Hamilton. She was reprising the role of Sarah Connor, a mother cursed with knowing that if she could keep her son alive, he would save Earth from an apocalyptic invasion of machines. Any Schwarzenegger movie featured buff bodies, but Hamilton had a harder job than most. She had to seem maternal enough to protect her son, yet vicious enough to keep him alive at any cost.

To pull it off, the actress trained to reduce her body to its barest muscular essence. On screen, her arms rippled like restless water and her stomach was armored by six-pack abs. She was, in sum, a starkly visual counterpoint to all the techno-wizardry unleashed by director James Cameron—one true thing amid the tinsel.

The stunning new look became part of the marketing for the movie. In an appearance on *Larry King Live*, Hamilton explained: "I worked out with a trainer six mornings a week, two to three hours every day, for most of last summer three months before we started to shoot, and then carried it on throughout the shoot. That was in the mornings. Then in the afternoons I worked with another coach learning guns and weapons and military skills and judo and all kinds of things to try to hone the internal body as well as the muscles."

How could audiences not notice? Writing in *The New York Times*, Janet Maslin observed: "Vicious and feral, showing off a bodybuilder's phenomenal muscle tone, Sarah says more about Cameron's taste for ferocious heroines ... than for the future state of women warriors." The look also provided a bold new direction for American women.

A nurse in Omaha might feel a little creepy imitating a Ms. Olympia. But Linda Hamilton still looked like the housewife next door, just a buffer version who made women everywhere reconsider what it meant to be powerful.

SAN DIEGO
September 13, 1991

As he reached the sixth anniversary of becoming the FDA's National Steroid Investigation Coordinator, it was beginning to dawn on Dennis Degan that he might not see a seventh. The old guard that had supported him was on its way out, and the new commissioner, David Kessler, was in the midst of a full-scale retreat from the steroid war. Instead of pouring resources into Degan's unit, Kessler was starting a new Office of Criminal Investigations to focus on things that were more central to the FDA's mission—like fraudulent drug applications or unsanitary restaurant conditions. Degan was given a chance to run it, but perhaps too stubbornly, turned down the invitation. He didn't want to change his focus or move his family to the nation's capital.

For a time, he thought he might have a role as a liaison between the FDA and DEA. But no one at the DEA seemed the least bit interested in him. A group of low-level "fact-finders" made a trip to his Detroit office to leaf through his 750,000 pages of files late in the summer. No one ever called back. His files still sat there, untouched.

Degan's anxiety increased when he proposed yet another expansion of his steroid beat, this time with an investigation to target the top 10 counterfeiting labs in the country. He had been successful in shutting down the major smuggling routes, but counterfeiters were picking up the slack. One guy he had busted was selling milky white horse penicillin as Winstrol, oblivious to the fact that anyone who was allergic to penicillin would go into anaphylactic shock after shooting it. But, as he would later recall, he was told by a superior in a telephone call: "You'll do no such thing."

He looked at the phone, dumbfounded. It was the first time in six years that he was told not to make a case.

THE 405 FREEWAY, CALIFORNIA
October 31, 1991

Some things get easier with experience, but for Dan Duchaine, being indicted wasn't one of them. Not knowing who might be waiting for him after his arrest, he grabbed his girlfriend, Shelley Harvey, and checked into the Oceana Hotel in Santa Monica, paying in cash. A few days into their stay, he woke from an afternoon nap, feeling strange. "What's the matter, baby?" she murmured. He couldn't exactly say. In fact, he couldn't say much of anything. When he tried talking, nothing came out. Harvey took him to the hospital, where they learned that, a month shy of his 39th birthday, he had just had a mild stroke.

Hypertension is one of the least-understood effects of polycystic kidney disease. Duchaine was still fit, still the rock star that Harvey had fallen in love with. But the stress of the trial was hastening the cystic deterioration of his kidneys. His blood pressure was through the roof and his hands had started to shake. Still, the two were making optimistic plans for the future. He saw them living quietly in London on a tree-lined street with kids.

Harvey, however, was still focused on the thing she had come to America to get—a body rock-hard enough for her to win the upcoming British bodybuilding championships. She was close. Spread across her arms, chest, and legs were 14 new pounds of muscle, ripped and ready to ripple under show lights. But this morning, after she had come back from a particularly strenuous workout, Duchaine suggested they take an afternoon break from training. As the sleek Shelby Cobra parked outside attested, he loved building custom cars and there was an auto show in Orange County that he wanted to check out. "It'll be a nice change of pace," he said. Happy to see that his spirits were good, she said, "Sure, Dan." Because the Cobra needed work, they hopped on his Honda scooter.

It was perfect weather and neither was wearing a helmet to stop the air from blowing freely through their hair. Harvey gripped Duchaine's waist as he made his way onto the 405 and grabbed tighter as he got the Honda up to 50 mph. Then, out of nowhere, her world changed inalterably. The bike's back tire blew out. Duchaine frantically tried to keep it upright but it skidded on its side into the median. Before he lost consciousness, the last thing he saw was Harvey about 50 feet away, a thick trickle of blood coming from her head.

By nightfall, Duchaine awoke in a nearby hospital. "Where's Shelley?" he asked. In a coma, came the answer.

It took three weeks and one surgery for doctors to bring Harvey out of her coma and relieve the swelling that flared in the back of her brain. Duchaine was by her bed when she opened her eyes, and when she asked for a mirror, he reluctantly handed one over. The reflection showed that her long blonde hair had been shaved off. "Was that really necessary?" she asked in a cracked whisper. "I just had my highlights done."

Despite her attempt to make light of the tragedy, it didn't take long to see that Harvey was never going to be the same person. While she would substantially recover in later years, friends who had known her as a vibrant woman saw a person with a starkly limited range of expression. After she had part of her scalp removed and replaced to stave off infection, one likened her to a robot. Still, Duchaine took care of her with obsession that bordered on penance.

Larry Wood, meanwhile, was hoping they could turn their upcoming case into a show trial, the kind that could make them symbols for a younger generation of amateur chemists. But Duchaine, who so many years ago would have jumped at the chance, shook his head. He didn't want to divert money from Harvey's care by hiring an expensive lawyer. Better to accept the services of a free court-appointed attorney, even one whose hands were full of a million other things.

By the start of 1992—with the trial just a few months off— the signs of strain were showing. Duchaine's once-black hair was clearly going grey and he was spending more hours in his easy chair watching TV. Harvey's mother had come to visit her ailing daughter for a brief time, and she and Duchaine weren't getting along. "You call yourself a Christian, but you're not," he yelled at her. "If you were, you'd forgive me."

One afternoon, John Romano came by to pick up a book and found Duchaine sitting in his easy chair, staring at the TV screen with his forefinger pressed against his lip. "Hey, Dan," he said casually. When Duchaine didn't respond, Romano thought, "Okay, he's in another weird mood."

He didn't consider that his friend might be having another stroke.

7

THE BIGGEST BELIEVERS
April 10, 1992 - May 14,1992

The Guru checked his necktie in the mirror outside of the federal courtroom. It was slightly crooked and he brought up his lame right arm in a frustrated attempt to fasten it. His hand just fumbled at the knot, making it worse.

His second trial was about a drug that was used by a cult of people who believed in prolonging life. Yet the man accused of peddling it was aging rapidly before everyone's eyes. Thanks to the two strokes and the stress of watching his girlfriend recover from brain surgery after the motorcycle accident, Duchaine—still not yet 40—seemed to have aged another 10 years. His thinning hair was completely grey now, and he had wads of loose skin hanging about his face. Friends who called him were greeted by an answering machine that told them to speak slowly because he needed time to write down their words. He looked like a rebel without any fight left in him.

Inside the jury room, federal prosecutor Mark Byrne made sure the jury didn't have much time to look upon the defendant sympathetically. "This case is about fraud and about greed," Byrne said in his opening statement. "You will hear evidence that the defendants Lawrence Wood, who calls himself a doctor, and Daniel Duchaine, who calls himself a steroid guru, were in the business of selling two dangerous drugs, GHB and clenbuterol. They were selling these drugs to bodybuilders, and telling the bodybuilders these drugs were safe and would help them bulk up. But you will hear testimony from medical doctors and scientists that both drugs have serious side effects and are not approved for any human use in the U.S."

Duchaine sat quietly as Wood's attorney passed on his chance to address the jury, and his own court-appointed attorney tried to split a few hairs. Yes, her client sent out misbranded drugs that were regulated by the FDA. But "what this case will not show is that a fraud was committed," she insisted.

In other words, the jury would have to decide whether they were looking at a couple of cagey drug dealers or two principled advocates.

This wasn't quite the narrow question it seemed. Outside the courtroom, a much larger war was brewing between the worlds of alternative and traditional healing. In reasserting the power of the FDA, David Kessler had declared war on the faux medicine men who were making outlandish health claims, and their minions who sold unapproved nostrums and potions.

Kessler saw them trying to take refuge under a 1990 federal law that allowed cereal companies to make certain claims about their products, and he wanted to close the loop before things got out of control. This trial, however, was showing the difficulties that lay ahead of him. Terms that once seemed so simple were turning out to be extremely complex and in need of clarification. For instance, what was a vitamin?

When an FDA investigator was called to the stand and asked to define it, he stammered. "Well, I don't know," he said, finally. "It doesn't have a definition by the FDA. Vitamins aren't regulated." The implicit suggestion was that GHB shouldn't be, either.

When the trial resumed on April 14, Byrne tried to rebut that notion by calling a researcher who had done a critical study at UCLA 30 years earlier, Dr. Wallace Winters.

"How does GHB compare to LSD?" Byrne asked.

"GHB and LSD produce the same initial effects of hallucinations," Winters began, "but GHB is capable of going beyond that state up all the way to seizure activity." He explained that "as we go up the hallucinary [sic] stage, we find the visual system increases. Colors look brighter, there are more complications in simple geometric patterns, and so on. As we increase the dose of GHB, we see a tremendous increase in both the auditory and visual response. It's more than twice as high as it is in the awake state."

"Why would that be?" asked Byrne.

"Because the central nervous system is not modulating or controlling sensory signals coming in. It has lost the ability to control the systems. And that state occurs just before the individual goes into seizure activity. During seizures and after, the nervous system essentially collapses."

Byrne was almost across the finish line. "I realize you've been talking about seizures and hallucinations, but what are the dangerous, harmful side effects that can occur?" he asked.

Winters shifted: "Well, one of the first dangerous effects is taking this drug and not knowing that these are the consequences of that action. Secondly, is the fact that this drug can produce cardiovascular and respiratory alterations ... profound seizure activity."

And there it was. That was the key element of the fraud claim: that these two quacks were selling something dangerous without disclosing its effects.

The work of repairing the damage fell to a witness Wood had

recruited specifically for the task, Dr. Andrew Weil. The burly Harvard-educated doctor lived in Tucson, where he ran a medical practice that was getting national attention for its holistic approach. A folksy physician, Weil anticipated the openness that ex-hippies-turned-suburbanites would have toward alternative remedies, and was profiting handsomely from it. *Time* magazine had recently profiled him, noting admiringly that he sent some patients to get acupuncture and others to an Indian shaman, but that he drew "the line at crystals therapy."

On the stand, Weil's job was to tear down Winters's testimony and he took to the task lustily. Going through his CV quickly—an undergraduate and medical degree from Harvard; a stint in the jungles of Latin America, where he took psychedelic mushrooms—Weil testified that he had prescribed GHB to a dozen of his patients in the last three or four years and knew of 300 articles on its effects.

"What is the consensus?" asked Wood's attorney, David Elden.

"The consensus, first of all, is that GHB is an outstandingly safe pharmacological agent," Weil answered.

"Is it a hallucinogenic drug?" Elden continued, circling closer.

"Absolutely not.... In fact, it has the opposite effect of a stimulant. It's a sedative drug."

"Now, have you read any studies by Dr. Winters?"

"I have read seven papers that Dr. Winters published."

"And comparing Dr. Winters's conclusions in those papers to general information that's out in the science journals, is he in the mainstream?"

"Absolutely not," Weil replied. Winters only did his research in cats and used "enormously toxic doses." Looking at one of the cat photographs, Weil said that the animal had received a dosage "at least 10 times higher" than a human would take. "I think it's impossible to determine hallucinatory states in animal research. I mean, if you even think about it, how do you tell when an animal is hallucinating? You know, animals can't tell you they are seeing dragons."

The choice for the jury was now clear: between the government, which said its defendants were selling poison, and a new-age doctor who testified that the Food and Drug Administration was hopelessly behind the times. With things so neatly framed, both defense attorneys decided to keep their clients off the stand.

As the jury was sent to deliberate, Wood was optimistic. "We're gonna win this, Dan," he said. But Duchaine was resigned to the inevitable, and it was a good thing. The jury quickly returned with its verdict: guilty.

Duchaine looked ahead, unblinking, as motions were made regarding sentencing and appeals. Once again, he had fought the government and once again, it had repaid him the way it always did.

LAKE OSWEGO, OREGON

May 14, 1992

Lyle Alzado hung his leg over the side of the bed and tried to pick it up. He had been playing this game with himself for a while now. Since he could no longer speak and could barely eat, it was one of the last ways for him to monitor how much life was left inside of him.

The cancer in his brain was moving too fast to stop. In Los Angeles, his doctor, Robert Huizenga, was resigned to the fact that there would be no miracles. And Alzado's friends had already said their goodbyes with two benefit dinners in his honor. The first was a botched affair to raise money for the mounting legal and medical bills. (His manager had rented a ballroom for a $500-a-plate dinner but wound up giving away so many complimentary invitations that it unraveled at the last minute.) It was some of his old friends from Gold's who, a month later, finally came through.

Alzado walked into the Venice Beach Marriott and was enveloped by O.J. Simpson, Marcus Allen, and hundreds of others who rushed to shake his slim, bony hand. Since his doctors had recently ended his chemotherapy, he was able to enjoy the stories that were told about him without constant waves of nausea and fatigue. Still, it was a bittersweet moment when Derrick Barton, the marketing director for Gold's, raised a glass to toast Alzado, proclaiming him the gym's official Sergeant-at-Arms. He had to be helped to the podium to thank everyone. His once-booming voice registered barely above a whisper.

Not long after that, Alzado was on a plane out of Los Angeles for good. It was his wife, Kathy, who told him that they needed to get out of town. She hated the way his ex-wives were meddling, and her insecurities about them gnawed at her. And there were the money issues. To hell with it all, Kathy thought. To hell with the negativity. She would just move him away from everything.

Their destination was her family home in Lake Oswego, near a University of Oregon hospital that was offering one last experimental treatment. It involved the use of concentrated sugars and tiny catheters to open up the blood vessels that formed a fence-like barrier around his brain, making it hard for cancer drugs to reach it. The doctor who pioneered the procedure had done it about 3,500 times, but he was still sober about the chances. "It's pretty late in the game," the nurse said when Lyle and Kathy arrived for a consultation. Alzado thanked the doctor. Then, staring at his wife of less than a year, he said that he wanted to try anyway.

As his latest movie, *Neon City*, was making its debut in Canada, Alzado quietly checked into the Oregon Health Sciences University hospital in Portland. For the first few days, he sat in a bed with an IV drip pumping fluids into his body. But he had underestimated how little resistance he had left. The chemotherapy that had bombarded his mothball-sized tumors decimated what was left of his strength.

His body was wracked by so many reactions that his doctors feared he might die at any moment.

Back on April 3, Alzado had celebrated his 43rd birthday, drifting in and out of consciousness in the intensive care ward. On one of the rare moments where he wasn't stuffed full of tubes, he motioned for Kathy to bend down. "I can't do this any more," he finally whispered into her ear.

Reluctantly, Kathy moved him out of the hospital, and back to her parents' home, where a hospital bed awaited him in the living room. That was where Alzado was now, dangling his leg over the side, trying to figure out how much strength he had left.

He couldn't pull it back up.

Not much longer now.

Because he could no longer speak, it would have been useless to ask Alzado if he really believed what he had said about the steroids being the cause of his cancer. But some of the regulars at Gold's had already reached their own conclusion. They were a band—a band of believers—bound by drug use that inspired all of the qualities that they prized: loyalty, secrecy, pride. Their bodies were the indisputable evidence that steroids worked, and in the vast majority of cases, worked well. They had all read the studies that declared steroids were dangerous and laughed at them. Dangerous? Look around the sports world. Look around Hollywood. Steroids were everywhere. Some of the doctors who worked out in Gold's were part of the club. Most had even written prescriptions for them. Many were *still* writing them.

They still loved Alzado. Fifteen years later, they would still tell stories about the way he beat up people as favors, hunted women like a pro, and pushed himself further than anyone they had ever seen. Yet there would also be a hint of betrayal in their words. In search of one last shot of celebrity, Alzado had violated—no, decimated—their code. At a moment when he no longer had football, no longer had fame, Alzado had found a way to be famous forever. He told

Americans that steroids were to blame for his death, and that they shouldn't make the same mistakes he did. But the believers didn't believe it for a second.

In the years to come, they would repeat third-hand rumors that Alzado liked to cruise Santa Monica Boulevard looking for boys, hoping to link his death to HIV. (Huizenga and all of Alzado's ex-wives insist that there was no truth to it.) They would point out that his mother also died of cancer, trying to suggest the cause of death may have been hereditary. And they would also point to the enormous amount of growth hormone that he took over the years, noting that studies suggest the drug can cause dormant cancers to grow.

But none of that mattered. Thanks to Alzado, the world was now convinced that steroids could kill.

He tried to move his leg again. How much did Alzado hear of what happened next? Did he hear the nurse by his bedside wake up his sleeping wife? "It won't be long now," she said. Did he hear Kathy running through the house, screaming uncontrollably? And did he hear what Kathy finally said when she calmed down?

"It's okay, Lyle, you can go now."

The nurse put two fingers over his eyelids and closed them. It was time for Lyle Alzado to stop running.

PART II

TAPPING THE VEIN
1992-2000

8

MORMON MONEY

May 17, 1992 - August 21, 1993

It wasn't exactly the shot at Fort Sumter, but for Loren Israelsen it was close. On May 6, 1992, flak-jacketed agents from the Food and Drug Administration approached the Kent, Washington, medical offices of Dr. Jonathan Wright and kicked in his door at 8:45 a.m. Once they were inside, they shouted to his staff to hold up their arms and do as they were told. When the clinic was secured, the agents carted away a truckload's worth of vitamins, patient records, and equipment.

Even before the raid, Israelsen, a Salt Lake City attorney and pro-supplement lobbyist, had regarded the FDA with considerable alarm. The new commissioner, David Kessler, might have abandoned the hunt for steroids, but the activist appointee was turning his attention to some of their spiritual cousins—the natural health aids produced by Israelsen's client, Utah's powerful, $700-million-a-year supplement industry.

The supplement industry was already on the run in the courts. It hadn't escaped anyone's notice that Dan Duchaine and Larry Wood had been convicted a month earlier for distributing GHB. The main question that trial had raised—what was a vitamin?—lay at the very center of the new war Israelsen was now fighting.

As he saw it, the FDA had an unfair stranglehold over wellness in America. In conjunction with the major drug companies, it controlled new drugs that were brought to market and how they were used. On his lobbying visits to Capitol Hill, Israelsen had insisted that supplements played a vital role in the healthcare equation. This was, after all, a time of rising health costs, managed care, and an overall feeling of holistic helplessness. With his soft Midwestern cadence, Israelsen had argued that supplements empowered people by giving them a chance to chart at least some of their own medical destiny.

To that end, Israelsen's job was to convince Congress that a tricky piece of legislation passed in 1990, the Nutrition Labeling and Education Act, did more harm than good. In broad terms, the act allowed food manufacturers to advertise certain health claims, so long as they could show "significant scientific agreement." That was easy enough when it came to asking a giant company like Kellogg to back up the claim that bran helped reduce the risk of some kinds of cancer. But vitamins and minerals were considered food, too. And, as Israelsen argued, it was unfair to make the mom-and-pop owner of a supplement company do an expensive study before they could say the extract from a yucca plant might help ease arthritis.

Recognizing that the law was imperfect, Congress shifted the matter back to the FDA, and for most of 1991 a task force met behind closed doors to hash out the issue. What they came up with was so contrary to what the supplement industry wanted that Kessler kept it under wraps. It concluded that vitamins and minerals needed to be regulated in the same way as food, which meant that supplement makers had to adhere to the standard of "significant scientific agreement" before they could make a health claim. The FDA's internal analysis conceded that mom-and-pop companies would have to invest in costly medical studies as well; that was just the price they would have to pay for doing business.

Israelsen had tried to find an opening for compromise when he visited the FDA's headquarters in Rockville, Maryland, in February 1992. But the reception he got was as chilly as the Washington weather. "If you don't like the rules," an official told him, "talk to Congress." As he walked out of the meeting and into a blustery wind, Israelsen thought the FDA was overplaying its hand. Now, after the Washington state raid, he was sure of it.

For one thing, the doctor who had been raided wasn't an outlaw like Dan Duchaine. He had a medical degree from the University of Michigan and patients who swore by him. "For those of us who want to get well without loading up on drugs, it's our right to do so," a retired real estate developer named Janice Barron told *The Seattle Times*. "I can't even express my outrage about this."

That was all Israelsen needed to hear. Go to Congress? Absolutely. And he would make sure everyone there knew about Ms. Barron, and the millions of Americans like her.

As to the question of whom to approach on Capitol Hill, it really wasn't a question at all. Orrin Hatch, the 58-year-old senator from Utah, was a loyal friend to the industry. He also worked out regularly and belonged to the Church of Latter-day Saints, many of whom believed that Mormon Scriptures encouraged the use of herbs as "God's medicine." He had even sold vitamins as a youth. And considering the small stake Hatch owned in a money-losing supplement company called Pharmics, Inc. (and the fact his son was working for an industry lobbyist), one might say that he was still selling them.

While Dr. Wright was fanning the flames[1]—insisting that the government had taken away his right to treat needy patients with

---

1 In 1995, the government dropped the case against Dr. Wright. No charges were filed and all medical records were returned.

arthritis, multiple sclerosis, and other afflictions—Israelsen worked with Senator Hatch to mold an industry-friendly bill. By June 11, it was finally ready. Grandly labeled the Health Freedom Act of 1992, the bill sought to allow supplement makers to advertise "the potency" of their products without fear of them being labeled drugs or triggering rigorous oversight.

Israelsen was at a conference in Arlington, Virginia, when the bill was introduced. As it happened, he was sitting next to a table of senior FDA officials whose conversation he was able to overhear. One had just received news of Hatch's introduction. "Don't worry," another said. "It won't go anywhere."

One reason for their certainty was the strong opposition that Hatch faced in the House. Representative Henry Waxman, a Southern California Democrat, had just introduced a bill attempting to strengthen Dennis Degan's successors at the FDA by allowing them to issue subpoenas and obtain civil penalties against those under its jurisdiction, including supplement makers who exaggerated the powers of their products.

Through the summer, Israelsen watched while the Health Freedom Act got caught in the political crossfire. The lobbyist was sure that he had tapped into some deep well of American values— some potent political force—but Congress had other things to think about, particularly a Presidential election. As he kept up his round of Washington appearances, Israelsen could see that he was still viewed as a special-interest lobbyist pushing a novelty measure for hicks and for hippies. So he took what he could get.

As the 102nd Congress wound down, the legislature imposed a freeze that effectively stopped the FDA from issuing any new regulations until December 1993.

Israelsen had until then to get his Act together.

BOULDER, COLORADO
July 1992

Of all the Arnoldistas who had drifted through Gold's Gym in the mid-1980s, Bill Phillips wasn't on anyone's most-likely-to-succeed list. Certainly, there was nothing to suggest that he would one day become a best-selling fitness author with more than four million books in print. A painfully quiet man with an unusually weak handshake, Phillips had been something of a Gold's wallflower. But he was a savant when it came to sensing trends and a certified genius at exploiting them.

That's what Phillips was doing with *Muscle Media 2000*, the magazine whose second issue he had just published. There could be little doubt that Phillips had read Jason Mathas's low-budget Venice newspaper, *Modern Bodybuilding*. Phillips's new magazine had the same attitude and its most controversial writer, Dan Duchaine.

In many ways, Phillips modeled himself on Duchaine. He had been a teenage bodybuilder in Denver who came to California to strike it big. When that didn't pan out, he returned to his native Colorado to study sports nutrition and start a newsletter inspired by the *Underground Steroid Handbook*. Over the next six years, Phillips published from his mother's basement, steadily building circulation by taking out ads in the larger muscle magazines, which built a mystique around him. Those ads touted the findings of a famed "Colorado sports medicine researcher named W.N. Phillips" and boasted testimonials from oddball characters such as "Leonid Ostepenko, the general secretary of the Soviet Union Bodybuilder's Federation." The burgeoning minimogul, of course, wanted to give the impression that W.N. Phillips was a wizened scientist and not a 28-year-old with a mullet.

Phillips could see that his industry was in a state of transition. Magazines such as Joe Weider's *Muscle & Fitness* might still be selling the fiction that everyday guys could attain larger-than-life bodies without drugs, but it was getting harder to ignore the nasty headlines from Washington about steroid raids and supplement busts. Even Dan Duchaine was heading to prison for dealing GHB. Phillips reasoned that the time was right for a new kind of guru for the gym world.

The editor's note in his second issue was a succinct statement of his intent: "These supplement companies and other power brokers honestly believe that they own this industry. And, in a way, they do. Most information providers can't afford to print anything that will piss off their big advertisers. Well, when advertisers like these approach me ... I tell them they can forget about it. Not only do I not need their whining and bitching about the editorial content of the magazine, but I don't want anything to do with their fraudulent garbage products."

It was a masterstroke of positioning: At the same time Phillips was establishing himself as an iconoclast, he was getting into the supplement game himself. He had recently been introduced to Newport Beach physician Scott Connelly, who had developed something that Phillips was sure he could sell, a protein and carbohydrate powder for postoperative patients who needed to put on muscle mass.

Phillips signed on to be the exclusive distributor of the product they called Met-Rx. He also put Connelly on the masthead of his magazine, swiftly dispensing with the promise he had just made to his readers.

THE BRONX, NEW YORK
September 4, 1992

The box score for Jose Canseco's debut in a Texas Rangers uniform read 0 for 4, with an RBI. But at least the win by the New York Yankees gave the press something to write about. The more they were focused on the field, the better for him.

Countless column inches were being devoted to the mystery of why the A's had suddenly, inexplicably, decided to break up Canseco's electrifying partnership with Mark McGwire. To be sure, they were an odd pair. The son of a manager for an oil company, Canseco had been drilled with self-doubt as a child. McGwire, meanwhile, was the product of an athletic family who seemed destined for stardom. The former lived out his life in tabloid style, the latter was a self-consciously private man who had married his first love, the batgirl of the team he played on at USC. But six years earlier, the general manager of the A's, Sandy Alderson, decided to bring them together in an experiment that would have profound implications on the game of baseball. It would also transform the steroid culture itself.

When it came to conventional notions of strength and size, Alderson was a heretic. Most ball clubs shunned weight lifting, repeating old maxims about size slowing down bat speed. Alderson believed that size mattered, especially with a game plan built on the long ball. One of his most important hires was an ex-A's infielder named Dave McKay, who treated the weight room like a temple. McKay began a conditioning program unlike any other in baseball, dragging his players out of bed in the mornings—even while they were on the road.

Not everybody agreed with his methods. As former A's DH Dave Parker would say: "If I got in at 3 a.m., I didn't want no one calling me until noon the next day." But McGwire and Canseco were willing converts.

McGwire had grown up in a family in which weight lifting was part of the lifestyle; his brother, Jay, competed professionally. Canseco, meanwhile, used the weight room much as Lyle Alzado had, to arm himself against a doubting father. Their effect on the A's clubhouse was palpable. It often looked like the backstage area of a Mr. Olympia contest, with the pair posing in the mirror, trying to out-buff each other. The duo, dubbed the Bash Brothers in the media, had helped the A's win 469 games and make three World

Series appearances (one of which led to a championship) since 1988. Which is why Canseco was sick about being sent packing.

To be sure, there were the off-field incidents: Those early career citations for speeding, and the arrest for gun possession. (He pleaded down to no contest on a misdemeanor weapons charge.) Then there was the incident in New York, in which the paparazzi had caught him coming out of Madonna's apartment. And of course there was the episode the past winter, when he had rammed his Porsche into his wife Esther's BMW.

But why trade him now, with the A's comfortably up by 7½ games in the AL West? And for whom? The Texas outfielder Rubén Sierra and two pitchers? Some reporters speculated that Alderson was looking ahead to 1993, when McGwire and 13 teammates would be eligible for free agency. Dumping Canseco now would shore up the pitching staff in the short term while giving the team longer-term salary flexibility.

Alderson may not have realized it, but the move also disposed of a time bomb. Canseco, who had become one of the richest players in the game in 1990 with a multi-year contract worth $23.5 million, was not shy about his steroid use. He started taking them in the minor leagues and openly recommended them when he arrived in Oakland, as he wrote in his 2005 autobiography, *Juiced*.

One of the people who claimed to have supplied Canseco was a Southern California gym rat named Curtis Wenzlaff. A personal trainer for an upscale gym in Fountain Valley, California, Wenzlaff was no hanger-on. He lived with, and worked for, the assistant to the A's president for community relations, Reggie Jackson.

The two met at Racketball World in 1988 and quickly began a friendship. Besides training Jackson, Wenzlaff worked at Jackson's Chevrolet dealership, opened a beeper store with a loan from him, and lived in his apartment on an on-and-off basis.

"Reggie knew everybody," Wenzlaff would tell the New York *Daily News* in 2005, explaining how he got inside the A's orbit. He attended parties where the A's gathered and was a frequent guest in Jackson's box. Through those connections, he met Canseco and, he would claim, began dealing to him. Wenzlaff also got to know McGwire, and would claim that he started delivering drugs to him, too. Notes that he showed the *Daily News* (and later, ESPN) pointed to a cocktail that included Winstrol V, two types of testosterone, and the veterinary steroid Equipoise. (In a 2005 interview with the *Daily News*, a McGwire spokesman refused to address the charges, saying simply, "We believe one should consider the sources of such allegations." While Canseco has been forthcoming about his steroid use, he has said he couldn't remember Wenzlaff.)

All of the above might have gone unnoticed, but for one unfortunate turn in Wenzlaff's life: he had found himself the subject of an FBI investigation.[2] An undercover agent had heard that Wenzlaff was dealing steroids and used an intermediary to broker an introduction. During a visit to Wenzlaff's home in January 1992, the agent noticed a framed photo of him with Canseco.

"I'm his trainer," Wenzlaff said proudly. "I put him on a couple of cycles."

The undercover acted impressed. He bought $2,000 worth of steroids that day and arranged for more buys, doubling the quantity in February and doubling it again in May. Hours before the A's were scheduled to take the field in Detroit on July 7, the undercover agent met Wenzlaff for a fourth time at the Guest Quarters Motel in Santa Monica. The agent said he was hungry and told Wenzlaff to order some room service. When a knock came at the door, the bodybuilder opened it to find a man in a trench coat. "Mr. Wenzlaff," he said, flashing an FBI badge, "You're under arrest."

---

2 FBI supervisor Greg Stejskal and undercover agent Bill Randall kept their probe confined to Michigan until they received a call from a supervisor at FBI headquarters in Washington, saying that an aide to President George H.W. Bush was inquiring about whether the FBI had any big steroid cases in the pipeline. As a result of the inquiry, Stejskal was given a green light to take the case national. He never learned the reason for the Bush Administration's sudden interest in steroids. But since Senator Biden was holding hearings at the time, it stands to reason that the president wanted to appear engaged with the issue. But it's also intriguing to note that his son George W. Bush was a managing general partner of Canseco's Texas Rangers at the time.

An indictment against Wenzlaff was unsealed on August 10. There was no mention of Canseco or McGwire, no public connection made to them at all. Whomever Wenzlaff had actually supplied, the government had decided to take the safe route by indicting the dealer but not pursuing his users, who, at most, would have faced a year in jail and most likely would have merely received probation.

It was an act of discretion that, despite the best of intentions, helped sustain a baseball-wide cover-up for at least another decade. An investigation might well have exposed other MLB players. It could have answered other mysteries that would remain unsolved years afterward, such as, did the Oakland organization know it had a dealer in its midst? Wenzlaff had at least a passing acquaintance with Alderson, and frequently sat beside Jackson in the stands.

Reggie Jackson, for his part, has said that he had no idea that his friend was dealing steroids—they were not in fashion when Reggie played—and Wenzlaff backs up the assertion. But Jackson had been around the game for quite a while. Did he not at least have suspicions?

And what about Wenzlaff's other clients? Years later, he would claim he had been supplying between 20 and 30 MLB players, along with 10 others from the NFL. He would fly to their homes, he said, with a few thousand dollars of Deca-Durabolin or Parabolan in vials he would wrap in tinfoil and stuff into shoes in his luggage. Yet he kept their names to himself.

LAS VEGAS
September 14, 1992

Dan Duchaine didn't want his girlfriend Shelley Harvey to live alone in Los Angeles while he did his second stint in prison. Too many creeps hung around Gold's, looking to prey on girls like her. It would be safer if she just returned home. So they both packed bags for very different places and took a taxi from Venice to Las Vegas. The five-hour ride had a funereal feel and when they finally arrived on the Strip, Duchaine tried to leaven it with a surprise. "Let's get married," he told Harvey. He bought her a sleeveless dress that showed off her arms and a bouquet of flowers, then told the cab driver to head to City Hall.

Not surprisingly, the wedding was ill-fated from the very start. After they had taken their vows and walked back outside, a passerby yelled "faggots," thinking that with her big biceps and buzz cut, Harvey was a man. Still in her wedding dress, she climbed back into the cab with Duchaine for the final leg of their trip together—the minimum-security prison on the Nellis Air Force base. Harvey walked her new husband to the office and waited for him to sign in. After a few minutes, he walked out with tears in his eyes. "It's time," he said. She turned away, sobbing too, and headed to the Vegas airport for the long flight back to London.

With all that he had been through, Duchaine was convinced their relationship could survive his latest prison term. "This is a *real* marriage," he wrote his sister, Sheila, as soon as he had settled into his new routine. "... Shelley and I plan on having twins *before* I get out of here. I get 'vacations' every three months. We're planning to extract two eggs from Shelley, fertilize them with my [frozen] sperm and re-implant them."

His optimism was tempered only by the fact that he had finally confronted what he had long been avoiding: "I got an ultrasound scan and confirmed that I have the polycystic kidney disease," he wrote to Sheila. He also told his sister about the stroke he had had before his trial. "No physical damage," he wrote, "but my speech and writing was hard and slurred for about eight weeks. All the tests couldn't figure out whether it was a clot (in the brain) or a burst blood vessel. I took [an] afternoon nap and when I got up I couldn't tell the time; speaking was impossible. Couldn't remember things while writing. I'm much better now."

The self-diagnosis was short lived. One night that October, Duchaine was rushed to the prison's infirmary with dangerously high blood pressure. At four in the morning, a decision was made to move him to the Federal Medical Center near Baton Rouge, a sprawling collection of buildings that happened to include a leading hospital for Hansen's disease, also known as leprosy.

"All the inmates are either sick or damaged—wheelchairs, missing limbs, etc.," he wrote darkly in another letter to Sheila. "Oh well, it's an adventure."

To get through, Duchaine continued to write for Bill Phillips's *Muscle Media*. The feds might have dumped him in a leper colony, but he would be damned if he would let that keep him silent. Shortly after Halloween, however, Duchaine was informed that he had also been slapped with a Central Inmate Monitoring Certificate. As he told his sister, "That means all my transfers, furloughs, half-way house visits, etc. have to be approved by the central prison bureau [in Washington, D.C.]. Basically, it's extra punishment because of my outspokenness."

DETROIT
February 20, 1993

Dennis Degan was perhaps the greatest bloodhound the FDA had ever known. Unfortunately, he couldn't pick up the scent of trouble in his own career.

Since the election of Bill Clinton as president of the United States, the ground had shifted under Degan's feet. Clinton was extending the term of his predecessor's FDA director, David Kessler, but instead of keeping the status quo, Kessler was undertaking a dramatic change. To be more responsive to the concerns of Congressional Democrats, Kessler had created a new Office of Criminal Investigations. This should have been good news for Degan, a sign that new resources were being poured into enforcement. But the man tapped to oversee it was a by-the-book ex-Secret Service agent who had little tolerance for Degan's seat-of-the-pants exploits. In the old days, Degan came and went as he pleased. Not anymore.

When no one from the new unit visited him in Detroit, Degan began to feel that he was being shunted aside. In early February, a retiring director whom Degan considered an ally, invited him to Rockville. Walk around, shake some hands, he was told. It might help. So Degan packed a bag and went. Deplaning at Washington's National Airport, he felt a sudden surge of hope. Maybe he had more support than he realized. Maybe it was just a matter of personalities. Sure, he was headstrong, but he was a loyalist. Everyone had to know how much of his life he had given to the war on steroids.

When he arrived in Rockville, Degan was introduced to the new investigations chief, and the two took the opportunity to go into an airless conference room for a talk. Though he didn't technically work for the Office of Criminal Investigations, it was made clear that Degan would not have much authority if he continued trying to work outside of it. The first question that was raised dealt with his independence: "Would you consider moving here, to Washington?"

Degan had been asked that very question six months ago and he had rejected the idea immediately—and brashly. "If I wanted to move to Washington, I'd have your job," he shot back. As soon as he said it, he regretted it. That was his frustration talking. But the mood was set. Each man was too wary of the other to reach any middle ground. After a half hour, the new chief got up to end the meeting. "I suppose I'll have to pick your brain," he said half-heartedly.

"Yeah, I suppose," Degan replied. And with that, he headed back home, no better for the trip and very possibly worse.

Degan buried himself in the case of a Mexican cancer doctor who was smuggling unapproved drugs over the border to his patients in the United States. It was just the kind of case that could make him forget his political troubles, a wide-ranging investigation with broad public health implications. He had gotten his old friend, the Assistant U.S. Attorney Phil Halpern, to work with him in San Diego and together they were generating enough leads to seek out two dozen search warrants in seven states.

While he was in the midst of typing one of the applications, Degan's office phone rang. It was a supervisor at FDA headquarters with some bad news: his office was being shut down. He had to hand all his files—including all the work on steroids—to the OCI and he would be reassigned shortly.

He put down the phone speechless. Wrap it up? Transfer his files? He asked Halpern to take the extraordinary step of flying to Washington to tell his bosses they couldn't suddenly yank him away from his pending work. Subsequent negotiations led to a compromise in which he was allowed to continue working on the Mexican cancer case. But it was a one-time exception. As far as headquarters went, he was in a bubble. In the long term, he was done. And he still had to turn over his files.

Degan was 50, still in the prime of life. He had prosecutors who swore by him and his instant recall of the informants, smugglers, dealers, or dopers who mattered. The names that didn't come to mind immediately were stored in the 750,000 pages of documents he had collected over the years. Now he was putting them in storage. He took some tape and sealed a few more boxes, then called building maintenance to cart away the first batch.

Over the next few years, Degan would come to work and look at the boxes gathering dust in a storage area. Eventually, they were destroyed. No one ever came to look at them. No one cared.

ROCKVILLE, MARYLAND

June 15, 1993

Despite considerable pressure, David Kessler was getting ready to release one of the most explosive documents in his office's history— his task force's report on supplements. The report's author, a deputy commissioner named Gary Dykstra, had been forced to cancel a speaking engagement because he had received death threats from industry activists who feared what might be in it. (Dykstra decided to give his speech via satellite instead.) Calls were coming into the FDA by the tens of thousands, and these weren't from kooks. They were Main Street Americans who had been galvanized into thinking that the FDA wanted to take away their vitamins.

Two months earlier, Senator Orrin Hatch had introduced a new bill to replace his ill-fated Health Freedom Act. Standing before the Senate, the gentleman from Utah told his colleagues: "We need to establish a regulatory structure that will encourage good health through the use of nutritional supplements while, at the same time, protecting consumers from unsafe products." He wanted to do that by turning the Nutrition Labeling and Education Act upside down. Instead of putting the onus on supplement makers to prove that their products were safe—as the labeling law required—Hatch wanted to place the burden on the FDA to show they were dangerous.

That concept went against every regulatory impulse in Kessler's body. He was still having nightmares about a rash of deaths that had been caused by a contaminated batch of an amino acid called L-tryptophan. And his desk was filled with hundreds of examples of supplement manufacturers who were making outrageous claims. Some even said their products could cure AIDS.

The time for quiet deliberation was over. He only had six months before a freeze on the current regulations expired. After that, both sides would have to suit up for war.

SALT LAKE CITY
August 21, 1993

Loren Israelsen heard about the task force report as soon as it was released. By the next morning, he had received no fewer than five copies from various sources.

If the Salt Lake attorney couldn't get what he wanted from the FDA, then this was the next best thing: a perfect present to fire up the troops, a document that proved he was right all along—the regulators in Washington really did want to ruin the supplement industry.

On the wall of his office hung a map of the United States with Congressional districts outlined in different colors. He knew that he had the Senate pretty well in hand, thanks to Orrin Hatch. But the House was another matter. The 1992 electoral landslide that continued the Democrats control also continued Henry Waxman's control of the House Energy and Commerce Committee's powerful subcommittee on health and the environment. Israelsen's only choice was to apply pressure. His electoral map for 1994 showed a dozen districts where Democrats might be vulnerable. As the summer wore on, he took his message to talk radio, and to anyone who might be listening at 2 a.m. in some small town in Texas.

Israelsen wasn't the only one trying to muster support. The supplement forces were a disparate lot, and his Utah contingent, with its roots deep in the Mormon culture, was only a small— albeit influential—part. The Council for Responsible Nutrition, the industry's venerable trade association, was keeping watch from Washington, D.C. And individual merchandisers, some with huge fortunes, were working in the trenches to do what they could do, too.

One, a tough-talking New Yorker named Gerry Kessler— head of the Nutritional Health Alliance and no relation to the FDA commissioner—managed to convince several high-profile Hollywood stars, including Whoopi Goldberg, James Coburn, and Mel Gibson, to appear in ads. In one, Gibson, who was about to make his directorial debut with *Man Without a Face*, was shown having his stately home invaded by a SWAT team from the FDA.

The commercial, which played repeatedly on television, added an element of glamour to what had previously been a niche issue. It also led to a national day of protest called Blackout Day. On Friday, August 13, health food stores were encouraged to place black crepe paper over shelves containing supplements that could soon be banned and tell anyone who tried to buy those products that they might not ever be able to if the FDA had its way. Phones were put on checkout counters so customers could call Congress to complain. Others were given stamps to send letters.

When he began the campaign, Israelsen had been the only one sounding an alarm. Now he wondered if things might be going too far. A few Congressmen had personally phoned him to complain that the calls coming into their offices were over the top; some included outright threats. He tried to strike a moderate tone. But his message to the public was unchanged:

Write your Congressman—your health depends on it.

9

THE PERFECT PITCH

May 1994 - October 1, 1994

GOLDEN, COLORADO

May 1994

Bill Phillips had great hopes about the two visitors who were flying in from California to see him. The mullet he had sported a few years ago was gone, replaced by a stylishly close-cropped haircut and the wardrobe of a man who was going places. He had a Rolex on his wrist and a red Lamborghini in the lot outside. He had also helped to sell $18 million worth of Met-Rx in 1993 and projections were even better for this year. Phillips had turned himself into such a celebrity that a photo in the January issue of *Muscle Media* had featured him with his arm around Playboy Playmate Anna Nicole Smith.

Not everyone thought Met-Rx was such a great product. Kim Wood, the strength coach for the Cincinnati Bengals, hired a consultant to do an analysis and was told that it was nothing more than a variation on a protein shake like Slim-Fast. It didn't matter. The smooth-talking Phillips drowned out the doubters in torrents of hype. Using the tough new steroid laws to his advantage, he positioned Met-Rx as a safe alternative, going so far as to offer a free month's supply to any student who sent him a blood test showing steroid use, a school ID, and a pledge to stay clean. Displaying a canny eye for grabbing headlines, he even convinced the strength coach of the Dallas Cowboys, Mike Woicik, to help him promote a "Steroid-Free Sports" stunt during Super Bowl XXVVIII in Atlanta.

One had to wonder whether Woicik, who was prominently featured in the next issue of *Muscle Media*, read the magazine carefully. The same issue in which he appeared carried stories about how to buy the steroid Equipoise through a veterinary supply catalog, how to build muscle with insulin, and where to get the latest experimental steroids, along with a Dan Duchaine column for female bodybuilders about how to avoid developing male characteristics while taking steroids.

One of the main functions of the magazine, however, was still selling Met-Rx. Phillips's capacity for hawking it seemed to know no bounds. He held contests for readers who sent before-and-after photos of themselves, ran wall-to-wall testimonials to its effectiveness, and, of course, supplied photos of his own rock-ribbed body. What his magazine didn't report on was the friction growing between him and Met-Rx's developer, Scott Connelly.

That explained the meeting he was having this morning with two supplement makers who were struggling to keep their small company afloat. They had supposedly stumbled on something new, something called creatine. What made the new powder unique was that it was actually so commonplace. Creatine is an amino acid manufactured in the body and found in red meat. Most doctors felt that people got all they needed from their diet. And since there was no evidence the body had the capacity to absorb extra amounts, the conventional wisdom was they wouldn't do any good.

But Anthony Almada, whom Phillips welcomed into his office,

was prepared to argue exactly the opposite. While leafing through journals at the University of California medical library in San Francisco, the biochemist found a Swedish study that reported on how concentrated doses of creatine got absorbed in human muscle tissue and stayed there. Almada claimed to be his own best test subject. After taking 20 grams a day, he insisted he had added 20 pounds to his dumbbell curls. With a friend, he invested $225 in a kilogram of creatine powder. Since that day in 1992, they had been marketing it under the name Phosphagen.

Phillips liked the way it sounded. He thought it had possibilities. He also liked their attitude. Almada and his partner, Ed Byrd, were hungry. (Byrd was especially so, since he had pleaded guilty to distributing GHB and was serving a five-year probation sentence.) But Phillips wasn't about to make the same mistake that he had made with Connelly by underselling himself. In fact, just yesterday he had called Byrd to suggest that maybe he shouldn't make the trip to Colorado after all. "I really don't think you have much," he said.

Byrd and Almada couldn't figure out if Phillips was trying to improve his negotiating posture, or if he was just a flake. No matter, they decided to make the trip anyway and now Phillips was giving them a guided tour of his offices. They were coolly designed in expensive chrome and the walls were lined with photos of the stars who had agreed to endorse Met-Rx—Troy Aikman and Sylvester Stallone.

The visitors couldn't help but be struck by how smoothly Phillips ran things. In one area, staffers were busily putting out *Muscle Media,* while in another, operators were taking orders for Met-Rx that were promptly filled at a loading bay in the back. Phillips quickly got down to business. They could have access to his well-oiled marketing machine in return for a 30 percent stake in their company, EAS. By the end of the day, all of their signatures were on the document.

ARLINGTON, TEXAS
August 11, 1994

Jose Canseco packed the things he had kept in his Texas Rangers locker into six small boxes and got ready for the trip back home to South Florida. The night before, he had been part of the Rangers' sixth loss in a row at Rangers Ballpark in Arlington, a 3-2 extra-inning embarrassment against Seattle. His team had spent most of July riding high. At one point, they were 12½ games up over his old club, the A's. But since then, they had been skidding like a hog on ice. The players were feuding amongst themselves and Canseco had been distracted enough by what he thought were bad calls at the plate to start videotaping his at-bats and showing them to umpires after games. In the meantime, the A's were on a roll, playing .615 ball—even with Mark McGwire out with a season-ending injury to his left heel.

That's what made the previous night's game so irritating. Canseco had missed a perfect chance to seal a win when he jammed his left ankle sliding back to first to beat a pick-off. Favoring his right leg, he wasn't able to score from second after a teammate hit a single to center. The Mariners wound up winning and the A's stayed within a game of Texas atop the AL West.

And with a work stoppage looming, Canseco didn't want the season to end now, not like this. After a couple of underperforming years, he was finally on his way back, one of a dozen players who were making the 1994 season one of the biggest surprises in MLB history. With a few months to go, he had hit 31 home runs, 12 off the torrid pace of Matt Williams, the league-leading third baseman for the San Francisco Giants, but still enough to be in the eternal conversation about threatening Roger Maris's single-season record of 61. There was a lot of talk about why—the lively ball theory was a favorite—but no one wanted to look too deeply. Surely not baseball itself.

Greg Stejskal, the FBI agent who had arrested the man claiming to be Canseco's supplier, would come across MLB's security chief, Kevin Hallinan, at an FBI conference in Quantico, Virginia, in a few weeks. Casually, he would mention the way he had tied Canseco to the indicted dealer, Curt Wenzlaff. Hallinan, according to Stejskal's recollection of the incident years later, would just shrug and ask what could he do? (The meeting would not be revealed publicly until the New York *Daily News* wrote about it in 2005.)

Clearly, baseball had more than steroid use to worry about. Of all the surprises that the season had produced, the biggest was the way players and owners seemed hell-bent on destroying the season by striking. A group of small-market teams, led by Milwaukee Brewers owner Bud Selig, wanted a salary cap to drive down salaries and were talking lockout to get it. A few hours earlier, Canseco got the word. The players union had voted to strike at midnight.

All around the league, players were going home to make tee times, reacquaint themselves with family, and hope that they could get back to business soon. Canseco, one of the loudest supporters of his union, personally stood to lose an estimated $24,044 for each day the strike dragged on. That was enough incentive for him to keep sharp. But he was a gym freak, a guy who would have pushed himself to his physical limits anyway. The strike was more significant for those players who suddenly found themselves without team trainers to keep them in shape. They were thrown out on their own, forced to find alternatives wherever they could, which usually meant local gyms. Weight gurus who normally couldn't get near a clubhouse were now sidling up to players, promising to help them keep their edge.

It was also a perfect storm for a supplement industry that was on the cusp of a radical change.

WASHINGTON, D.C.

August 1994

In the dog days of August, Loren Israelsen watched a third version of his beleaguered supplement bill finally pass through the Senate. Ted Kennedy, once an implacable foe of the legislation, offered his endorsement after its supporters agreed to a provision that gave the Secretary of Health emergency power to seize supplements that posed "an imminent and substantial public health hazard" in the event that the FDA didn't have the authority to do so.

For Israelsen, it was a small price to pay for a bill that offered plenty of other benefits. If this version of the bill passed, supplement makers would soon have the legal right to make claims about how their products affected the "structure or function" of the body. Just as important, the bill gave supplement sellers the right to display "truthful and balanced" medical information, so long as it didn't "promote any specific product or brand," and was "maintained in a location which is physically separate from the products," meaning a nearby countertop or bookshelf.

The changes were enough to get all members of the Senate to sign on. Yet there was a hint of intrigue and mischief to the way it was passed. The Senate chamber was nearly empty when Orrin Hatch brought it up for a vote in the wee hours of August 13. Under the rules of unanimous consent, all it took to pass was two senators who were barely awake to vote yes.

But the deft parliamentary maneuver only achieved half of what Israelsen needed. There was still a brick wall in the House, where the 10-term congressman Henry Waxman stood in the way, vowing to keep the bill bottled up in his subcommittee. Senator Hatch acknowledged as much in brief remarks that he made for the Congressional record. "I want to make very clear," he said, "that we recognize that there will be no final bill without the participation of our House colleagues."

If Waxman didn't already know how well-organized the supplement forces were, he got a taste of their zeal during the Congressional recess, when he went home to run for re-election and hold town hall meetings across his Los Angeles district. Supplement bill supporters quickly turned them into showdowns. Even the Hollywood set was turning against him. At a trade show in central Florida, the silver-haired actor James Coburn created a frenzy among hundreds of vitamin sellers by folding his hands into a 45-degree angle to show how he was once crippled by arthritis, and then unfolding them to show how liver pills had helped cure him. With his silkily rumbling voice, he shouted, "It's you, it's me, it's us against the FDA."

The next week, Israelsen got a call from a Waxman aide whom he had been trying to meet with for months. "I'll give you 20 minutes tomorrow," he was told. He arrived the following day, drenched in sweat from a cab ride that wasn't air-conditioned. As he was led to the aide's office, he put on his best poker face.

Israelsen felt the tide was turning in his direction, but he had to be practical. Many of his supporters were close to exhaustion. How often could he ask them to call their congressman or take part in a national protest? They had done their job. Now he had to do his. He had to get the bill passed.

As he strode into the House office of Waxman's subcommittee counsel, William Schultz, Israelsen extended his hand. "I really want to work with you on this," he said.

GOLDEN, COLORADO
September 1994

The fax that came through Anthony Almada's home machine made his head spin. Bill Phillips was calmly anticipating that they would do $9 million in creatine sales by the end of the year—nearly 20 times what they had earned the year before.

Creatine was all over *Muscle Media*. Almada had to look no further than the second page of the current issue, where a photo of Phosphagen resided at the top of the table of contents. The EAS product was also the focus of Phillips's ever-expanding direct mail operation. One piece he had just sent out featured a man dressed to look like an inmate standing behind bars, claiming that he had found a secret weapon that was just as good as steroids. The ad was a shrewd nod to the reality that most gym rats knew someone who had been arrested under the tough new steroid distribution laws and were looking for the next big thing.

But Phillips understood that those strategies alone wouldn't help him reach his sales targets. Which was why he was in the midst of another subtle shift in his business model. According to the editor's letter that would appear in his next issue, Phillips had polled his readers and discovered some interesting things about their desires. First, they had no use for coverage of bodybuilding contests. Rather, they wanted advice on practical things: nutrition, exercise and, yes, supplements.

Admittedly, these were the nuances of a niche market. And yet, Phillips was clearly on to something. The divide between average Americans and Arnoldistas was narrowing. It wasn't anywhere near as great as it was in the early days at Gold's, when some regulars stole cars and turned tricks to support their steroid habits. Muscular fashion was entering the mainstream. Gold's was up to 400 franchised locations and was now entering the soft drink market. And Arnold himself was leading the President's fitness counsel.

Phillips was simply anticipating the coming tide. Everything told him that all these people were just waiting to be led by someone who didn't look like a 'roided-up Mr. Olympia. That was the beauty of the contests he was running in *Muscle Media*, where he published readers' before-and-after photos. It democratized body image.

Not surprisingly, Phillips was stirring up jealousies among his rivals. Joe Weider's *Muscle & Fitness* had given him a broadside over the summer with an article entitled "The Anatomy of Misleading Ads—The Great Creatine Shell Game," claiming that creatine was ineffective and using science to bolster that claim. (Almada responded to the magazine's charges in *Muscle Media* with an earnest defense entitled "Setting the Record Straight" in which he refuted the science in *Muscle & Fitness*.)

But so what? Let Joe Weider keep running those creepy contests where the entrants were now grotesquely huge. Bill Phillips was staking out a more accessible future.

WASHINGTON, D.C.

October 1, 1994

Loren Israelsen was glad he had brought a sandwich. Because once the thick door closed on the conference room in the Rayburn House Office Building, the rules were laid down firmly: Leave and you don't get back inside.

Through late August and mid-September, he had been having nearly daily meetings with Henry Waxman's aides, trying to find common ground on something, anything. There were a few gains, but no movement on the central issue: Waxman, who had had an up-close look at how far the supplement people would go and was deeply distrustful of them, wanted to empower the FDA to regulate their claims before their products went on sale. Orrin Hatch, meanwhile, saw "pre-market approval" as the thing that stood in front of his holy grail. To pressure Waxman, he had gone to a trade show in Baltimore to rally his supporters. Write your Congressmen, he told them. "The time is now!"

But the last minute flurry of petitions had no effect. Representative Bill Richardson, the New Mexico Democrat who was sponsoring the House bill on Waxman's desk, couldn't sway his California colleague. "This isn't the Senate and I'm no miracle worker," Richardson told Israelsen.

By mid-September, Senator Hatch glumly addressed a meeting of about two dozen industry people to say that the effort appeared dead. "We did our best, and we'll come back to try next year," he told them. In politics, however, there's always one last card to play. And Hatch played his by sending Waxman the final version of the bill with all the latest revisions. "If it's going to die," he told Israelsen, "let it die in their hands, not ours." At least that way, Hatch reasoned, their side would be the ones to pay a political price.

With one week to go before the session ended, Senator Hatch made his appeal to John Dingell, chairman of the committee that oversaw Waxman's subcommittee. Couldn't they make one more attempt? All agreed to give it a try, so now Israelsen found himself in the Rayburn Building, spending his Saturday breathing stale air and hoping it might be freshened by a whiff of success.

As the day progressed, Waxman's camp seemed to be compromising on some key points, including one Waxman had seemed resistant to: letting supplement makers sell products without prior FDA approval. The bill was a grab bag of goodies for which Israelsen had been fighting for over three years. It allowed supplement makers to make claims about how their products affected the body's structure and function—a sticking point for the FDA—and allowed stores to display certain medical literature, increasing the air of authority around products such as bee pollen. Finally, any supplement that was on the market before October 15, 1994, could stay on the market, but the FDA had to be informed within 75 days if it had been chemically altered.

As the meeting broke at the end of the day, Israelsen couldn't help but feel that the whole exercise had been a little too easy. He turned to another attorney who had been intimately involved in the talks and said, "I hope we're not being set up."

The following Thursday, the House easily passed the new bill. That meant there was just one more hurdle: sending it back to the Senate for the final legislative step. Israelsen barely slept that night and spent all day Friday huddled over the phones. That evening, Hatch assured him they were now, gloriously, at the end of their road. But one bill after another was coming up for a vote, and with the clock nearly striking midnight, there was still no action. An aide kept calling a hotline to see if any holds had been placed on the bill. (According to the Senate's rules, it took only one senator to place a hold on a bill and the whole thing was dead.) Just before midnight, they got the news. Howard Metzenbaum, the retiring Democrat from Ohio, had done just that.

Israelsen slapped his hands together so hard that they stung. On the Senate's floor, Orrin Hatch was also in a rage. He cornered Metzenbaum to ask what the hell was going on. If this was the way he was going to act, Hatch wasn't without recourse. He intended on holding up the nominations of several federal judges whose confirmations were also pending that night. A deal was hurriedly worked out and at 12:24 a.m., the bill was finally called. The Dietary Supplement Health and Education Act of 1994 (DSHEA) passed by unanimous consent.

Loren Israelsen had spent years imagining what he would feel like when this moment came. But now that it was here, he felt too drained to celebrate. Handshakes and hugs gave way to yawns, and he told his colleagues that he would see them the next day for a victory postmortem.

He walked into the early hours of the fall morning and strode the few blocks to his hotel, then went to his room and collapsed on the bed. He flicked on the remote to watch the DSHEA wrap-up on C-Span as if it were a postgame show for the Super Bowl. Then he rubbed his head wearily.

"Now we have to show that we deserve what we got," he thought. "Otherwise, our critics are going to crucify us."

10

SOLACE AND SEX
February 27, 1995 - August 31, 1996

SAN DIEGO

February 27, 1995

John Romano pulled up to the arrivals gate at the San Diego airport in a white Econoline van and threw open the door for Dan Duchaine. "You look like hell," Romano said, clearing the way for Duchaine to climb into the front seat.

Duchaine's health had declined precipitously in the last year. After he had finished serving his time on the GHB case in June, he was re-incarcerated on a separate charge for violating his probation from the 1987 steroid case. That meant a change from the prison hospital in Louisiana to a federal correctional center in Fort Worth. But almost as soon as he arrived, he was shipped to the prison's osteopathic medical center for a renal ultrasound test.

The news about his kidneys wasn't good. The cysts were slowly growing. In September, he had suffered another stroke, requiring an arteriolar angioplasty procedure to open narrowing arteries in his brain. A subsequent Bureau of Prisons health report noted that, due to the hypertension, Duchaine had to be sheltered from the sun and cold. In perhaps the ultimate indignity, it also noted that he could not lift more than 25 pounds, so he was given a work assignment in the prison's "leisure library."

Romano also noticed that Duchaine's coloring was pallid and that his jeans hung loosely off his hips. His skin was pinched around his eyes, making them seem more sad than hard. Dan's rat-a-tat pattern of speech was also gone, too, replaced by a painfully slow delivery. "I ... know ... exactly ... what I ... want ... to do tonight," he said as they drove out the airport exit and onto North Harbor Drive.

The worst thing about prison for Duchaine had been the food. And that evening, he made a reservation at an Italian restaurant in San Diego he had been dreaming about for months. The menu was a revelation and for the wine, he chose one of his favorites, a De Loach Vineyard Zinfandel. It was a dry, complex wine and when it came, he put it to his lips expectantly. Yet after the first swallow, nothing registered on his tongue. He sipped again, this time more determined. Same thing. Then again. And again. And again. Finally, the reality sank in. It wasn't the prison food that had had no taste. The strokes had robbed him of that sense. All the time he had spent waiting for that gourmet meal had been a cruel tease.

As it turned out, so was the prospect of his reunion with his wife, Shelley. She had visited him twice in prison, ignoring the advice of her London doctors. But once they were in each other's company, it was obvious that the things they talked about in their letters—the house on a tree-lined block, the kids—was a distant possibility now. Shelley, still trying to recover from the brain damage of her accident, walked around frightened and disoriented. How could she take care of a child when she often couldn't take care of herself?

"I'm such a bad person. That's why you want to leave me," Duchaine told her. "No," she replied. "I just don't feel safe here in America, Dan." One day after speaking with her on the phone, he turned to Romano and quietly said, "Well, I guess that's it. She's not coming."

Instead, Duchaine turned to old friends for solace and sex, among them a Gold's Gym regular, Sandra Blackie. He asked her if he could take her out to dinner in San Diego one night and she eagerly agreed. Blackie remembered the old Dan Duchaine, the one who mixed the quiet confidence of a professor with the deviant twinkle of child. She remembered the way his body seemed oddly sexual, how it felt to be held in his powerful arms, or to slip her arms around his 19-inch neck. And how he used to be able to say so much without saying anything just by moving the lines of his forehead. But that man wasn't there anymore. Like Romano, she saw Duchaine for what he was now: older, paunchier, balder. Even the old twinkle seemed more desperate than dangerous.

After their meal, she and Duchaine went back to her place and he pulled a videotape from his coat. It was gay porn. She slipped it into her VCR and Duchaine watched a bodybuilder they both knew, blindfolded and being sodomized by another man.

"I don't know if we should be watching this," Blackie said, turning it off. Duchaine looked at her blankly. "Well," he said, disappointed. "I've been in jail for a while. A blowjob would be good."

Blackie let out a sigh. "Okay," she replied. "But this is a one-time deal, Dan. I've moved on from the old days."

Duchaine had to move on as well. He had admitted as much in a column that appeared in the January 1995 issue of *Muscle Media*. "Have you gone soft on steroids?" asked a reader who hadn't known that he had been in prison. "I've been away from the frontline of the bodybuilding chemical wars for close to two years," he wrote. "However, I don't think things have changed much.... To be blunt, anabolic steroids at the athletic level are not all that interesting to me anymore."

Dan Duchaine wanted a new challenge. And he found it in Orrin Hatch's DSHEA.

CONCORD, CALIFORNIA
February 1995

Mike Zumpano sat next to Mark McGwire in the conference room of his company, Champion Nutrition, and marveled at the size of the slugger's legs. Baseball players weren't supposed to be built like this. As the Philadelphia Phillie John Kruk once famously remarked to a woman who saw him smoking, "I'm not an athlete, lady, I'm a baseball player." But McGwire, *he* was an athlete.

McGwire was visiting Zumpano on the advice of his younger brother, Jay. During the last two seasons in which he was injured more often than not, McGwire moved to Northern California to live with Jay in a place near Zumpano. The brothers looked so much alike that they were often mistaken for twins, but it was more than just looks that bound them. Jay, an aspiring bodybuilder and personal trainer, was deep in the supplement business. As reporter Tom Farrey noted in a 1994 article in *The Seattle Times,* Jay had a stake in a company that sold supplements with names that sounded just like steroids and growth hormones—Anabol and GH releaser—and enlisted McGwire to help advertise them. By 1995, Mark McGwire was already enough of an expert to know the difference between Dianabol and the provocatively named products his brother sold.

But Jay was no longer involved with that company, and he was looking to connect his brother with another supplement supplier, which is why he brought McGwire to Concord. If Mike Zumpano had a suspicion about how McGwire got to be his current size, he didn't bring it up. Instead, he offered him a check for $50,000 and asked McGwire if he would endorse Champion's products.

Mark McGwire waved the offer away. "I don't want your money," he said. "Just give me all the supplements that I need."

The answer surprised Zumpano, but he caught himself. Was McGwire doing a favor for his brother? Or perhaps he was one step ahead of Zumpano. Maybe he needed this kind of an arrangement so no one would question where—or how—he got his physique. No matter. Zumpano was thrilled to have him on board. And McGwire was feeling healthy for the first time in three years and looking forward to a great season.

LAKEWOOD, COLORADO

April 15, 1995

As Anthony Almada piloted his new Ferrari to work, he couldn't believe how fast things were happening. Having already received positive test results showing that creatine helped replenish adenosine triphosphate (ATP)—a protein stored in muscles and burned for energy during workouts, Almada arranged for a professor at the University of Memphis to study other "real world" benefits. When the professor reported that creatine helped in performance testing by as much as 40 percent, his partner Bill Phillips went into hyperdrive.

He got himself invited to the Denver Broncos' training camp and sold the strength coach on the notion that extra ATP would help his players be quicker off the line of scrimmage. It wasn't long before half the teams in the NFL (as well as teams in Major League Baseball) were using it.

Pulling into his parking lot, Almada felt slightly giddy about the success. He had 30 percent of a company that was spitting out money like a broken slot machine, and a slew of new ideas, like mixing creatine with vitamins and minerals for a one-stop muscle gainer. Almada may not have liked Colorado much—he was a die-hard surfer and still went back to his place in Santa Cruz on weekends—but as the Ferrari he had just bought proved, it was hard to argue with success.

As he sat down at his desk, Almada saw a fax waiting for him from Phillips. The memo line was typical Bill: "Offer of a lifetime." Phillips's e-mail had nothing to do with promoting one of their products, however. "I think I want to move in a certain direction," Phillips wrote. He wanted to pay his partners $1 million to leave the company and if they weren't interested, then he was prepared to move his considerable marketing machine elsewhere.

Almada was floored. A million dollars? With all that EAS was pulling down, that was an insult. To find out what was actually behind the offer, Almada invited Phillips to his office in Lakewood for lunch. "It seems that you want full control, Bill," he said.

Years later, he could still remember the way Phillips replied with a soft whisper, "Yes I do."

TIJUANA, MEXICO
November 1995

"Get yourself a stack of pesos and put them on the bar," Dan Duchaine told the man on the barstool next to him. If there was one thing that became evident since Duchaine's release from prison, it was that he needed access to the new minds of his business. The young Bostonian hoisting a beer beside him, Bruce Kneller, was just what The Guru ordered.

Kneller was a registered nurse who grew up reading Duchaine's articles. While Duchaine was in prison, Kneller saw one of his columns and disagreed with a conclusion, sending a stack of medical literature to back up his point. Duchaine surprised him with a letter back that asked him to become The Guru's newest research assistant.

Their medical conversations ran late into many nights. But the one place Kneller couldn't rival Duchaine was in his lust for life's darker side. When he visited his new boss in San Diego, Kneller was greeted by the suggestion that they go carousing over the border in Mexico. They drove into Tijuana, then parked Duchaine's van and walked into a world of bustling alleys bathed by half-lit neon signs offering every manner of vice to cash-carrying Americans.

Pharmacies advertised steroids in their windows. Bars advertised far more than that. Duchaine grabbed Kneller by the elbow and followed two men through a nondescript door. Kneller was almost relieved to see that it was just a strip joint. They grabbed a seat and he ordered a round of beers. It was then that Duchaine told him to get a four-inch-high stack of pesos.

"Why?" he asked.

"You'll see."

Kneller did as he was told, and a stripper dancing atop the bar came by, eyeing the coins. Parking herself in front of him, she knelt down so that her buttocks touched the bar and, to Kneller's astonishment, sucked up the stack. Duchaine patted Kneller on the back. "You ain't seen nothing yet."

Almost on cue, the lights went down and the crowd looked over to a rickety stage where a donkey was trotted out on one end and a naked woman brought out on the other. As the woman lay down, the donkey was brought to her. Over the next few minutes, she proceeded to fellate the animal until it sprayed across her face. Kneller nearly fell off his chair in revulsion. Duchaine threw his head back and just laughed. Slapping Kneller, he said, "*Now* you'll have something to tell your Boston friends about."

There was more to the weekend. Back in Carlsbad, California, Duchaine had gotten Kneller drunk and hooked him up with a porn star. But by the time Kneller was ready to fly home, he had the feeling that it wasn't healthy to spend too much time around Dan Duchaine. The drug use, the endless women who offered their bodies up to him as experiments, the stints in prison, all the shady people he hung out with—maybe no one could have escaped all that with their psyche unscathed. But Duchaine seemed a bit *too* enamored of his demimonde. While being around him could be electric, it could also be toxic. Look at what had happened to his wife Shelley Harvey, and the countless women who had adverse reactions to his advice. Too many bad things happened to too many people who trusted Dan Duchaine.

Perhaps the toxic lifestyle was a reaction to what was happening inside of Duchaine—to the kidney disease that was slowly destroying his body. Maybe he sensed that he wasn't going to have to live with the consequences of his actions for long, so what the hell? Duchaine went to Mexico for a hair transplant to cover up the bald patch on the back of his head and got the baggy skin under his eyes lifted. But there was no mistaking the clock silently ticking inside the 43-year-old—the cysts expanding across his liver, pushing away the healthy tissue just as he was pushing away the healthy things in his life.

Through the fall of 1995, Duchaine dove back into being The Guru, although this time with a twist. Now that he felt truly unshackled, he wanted to write about his life, not hide behind his advice columns anymore. He wanted to show the world what he had shown Kneller—that all the wannabes could try to copy him, but none of them could stand to live the same reckless way that he did. He proved it in the November 1995 issue of *Muscle Media* with a new column he dubbed The Rant. For his first subject, Duchaine tackled the men who liked to pay female bodybuilders to wrestle with them or undress, otherwise known as "schmoes." Describing them with a sharp, unforgiving eye, he wrote:

> *Schmoes. Female bodybuilder worshipers. Loners. Not dangerous looking. Physically weak and begging to be domi-nated. Always lurking around bodybuilding shows. Most are near-broke. Take pictures with an Instamatic camera with a flashcube.*
>
> *One of the early female bodybuilders, who's still a stripper in Alaska, coined the term. It's probably some Jewish/ Yiddish term and shouldn't be applicable to these groupies, but somehow the name stuck. In other subcultures, you'll find opera-diva worshipers or fashion-model worshipers or*

ballet adulation. So it shouldn't be any surprise that schmoes
exist in female bodybuilding.

Duchaine was also eager to prove that he could keep up with all the new products being peddled under DSHEA. One of his new ideas involved pouring high doses of ephedrine—a molecular cousin of amphetamine derived from ma huang, an herb used in Chinese medicine—into a fruity Kool-Aid-like drink.

David Jenkins, his old steroid-smuggling buddy, had a supplement company called Next Nutrition that was based near where Duchaine was living in Carlsbad. Duchaine shared the recipe with him and after mixing up a batch in his basement, Jenkins decided that it tasted like a hit. He started selling it under the name Ultimate Orange with ads that tantalizingly warned it wasn't for "every Pencil-Necked Ding Dong in your gym."

Duchaine had no problem selling legal speed. After all, ephedrine was the least of what he put in other people's bodies. But he felt differently about steroids now. Although DSHEA had opened all sorts of doors, he still had nightmares about the feds knocking down his. If someone wanted to pick up his steroid torch, they were welcome to it.

SAN FRANCISCO
February 1996

Stan Antosh had only spoken to Dan Duchaine a handful of times, but their lives intertwined in a surprising number of ways. The son of a wealthy inventor and civil engineer, Antosh grew up in the farm country of Illinois, near Duchaine's old smuggling partner William Dillon. After studying accounting at the University of Iowa and the University of Texas, Antosh briefly owned a bar and grill near his family home, then decided to move to San Francisco. Broke but having a blast, he was working as a personal trainer and sleeping in the back of his station wagon when an acquaintance gave him a bottle of GHB. Antosh tried it and discovered that it produced the most beautiful four-hour burst of sleep he had ever experienced. Then one evening after he had taken his regular two-gram dose, he received a phone call that forced him to stay up late. The longer he fought off sleep, the woozier he became. As the call wore on, Antosh realized he had stumbled onto what club kids around San Francisco would soon realize: GHB produced a wicked high.

Antosh began buying GHB in bulk and advertising it as a cure-all for everything from impotence to depression, and even some cancers. At the suggestion of one of his customers—the life extension disciple Larry Wood—he also sent $1,800 worth of GHB to Duchaine and encouraged him to write about it. From March to October 1990, business was so good that Antosh slapped 65,000 labels on bottles. But in November of that year, California banned sales of the drug and Antosh had to go underground, using fake names while doing a cash business over pay phones.

Business continued to be brisk—perhaps too brisk. He was making tens of thousands of dollars a month and using so much of his own product with a girlfriend, she had to be hospitalized for a nervous breakdown. In 1991, he also got into the manufacturing end with his supplier, Mark Thierman, by setting up clandestine labs on the outskirts of Tucson. The danger of the business hit home when an employee who was using acetone, a highly flammable drying agent, left some by an open stove and triggered a massive explosion. The worker had the presence of mind to take his wallet before he fled so the feds wouldn't trace the lab to its real owners, and he delayed getting treated for his burns.

Astoundingly, Antosh decided the accident was just a minor setback. He and Thierman created another lab, and even more astoundingly, that place blew up, too. The person responsible for the second accident fled to Alaska rather than answer to feds who were drawn to the flames. This time, however, the ensuing investigation exposed Antosh and he was indicted on charges of running an unregistered drug-manufacturing facility and introducing misbranded drugs into interstate commerce, among other offenses.

Antosh had spent every day since studying borrowed law books for his trial. On this evening, though, he decided he needed a break. He put his textbook down, rubbed his tabby, Monroe, and grabbed a copy of the new supplement law that Congress had recently passed.

DSHEA was a cornucopia of regulatory treats for a chemical entrepreneur. That much was clear. But one thing stood out. It was the language that said a supplement was legal if its main ingredient was found in nature. Hell, he thought, you digest all kinds of cattle hormones when you eat red meat, and some of them metabolize into testosterone. All he had to do was find a chemical that seemed innocuous in nature, but did a metabolic magic trick once digested by turning into testosterone. Surely there had to be something like that. And if he was lucky enough to find it first, he would make millions. Or at least enough to pay his legal bills.

It was a perfect trade-off: One unregulated drug would be used to get him out of the trouble caused by another.

BOSTON

May 17, 1996

Pounding his glove in left field at Fenway Park, Jose Canseco watched Jason Giambi step up to the plate for the Oakland A's. Canseco didn't know much about Giambi, who had been called up from the minors the year before, other than the fact that he had become the new protégé of Mark McGwire. They partied together, took batting practice together, and shared the secrets of the game. Even from left field, Canseco could see that the 25-year-old Giambi was learning more than hitting. His body looked twice as large as Canseco remembered from the prior summer.

As Red Sox pitcher Tim Wakefield delivered a pitch, Giambi sent it sailing up toward centerfield. Gone. It was the 4,000th home run in Oakland A's history, and the A's cleared out of the visitor's dugout to help Giambi celebrate. Though he was in a Boston uniform, Canseco deserved to be part of the celebration. After all, he had hit 257 home runs for the A's—44 of them during his MVP year of 1991, when soon-to-be-indicted Curtis Wenzlaff claimed he had provided Canseco with steroids. (In an ironic twist, Wenzlaff's part-time employer, Reggie Jackson, had started the A's record on April 10, 1968 by hitting the first home run in Oakland's history.)

Now McGwire was following Giambi to the plate, and Canseco, his former Bash Brother, was readying himself in the outfield. McGwire was also on a tear, having reached base in each of his last 19 games. Wakefield tried to shake off the prior home run and served up one of his knuckleballs. But there wasn't enough movement on it. McGwire planted, turned, and sent it flying toward the Green Monster and right over Canseco's head.

As it happened, the A's lost in the 11th inning after taking an early 2-0 lead. But this was the fourth time so far this season that Giambi and McGwire had homered in the same game, and the pressroom was filled with questions for the new Bash Brothers. McGwire wasn't talking to the media, but Giambi was happy to supply a reason for their prodigious production. "It's the same restaurants, going to lunch together. That's it," Giambi said with a wink. "I'll look at the menu, and if it has hits in it...."

To a press corps that wasn't looking closely at answers, it was as good an explanation as any.

SAN FRANCISCO
August 1996

As the summer of 1996 progressed, Stan Antosh was beginning to feel that his hunch about GHB would pay off, thanks in large part to a recommendation that Dan Duchaine had made. Duchaine suggested that Antosh hire a creative chemist he knew named Patrick Arnold.

Like Duchaine, Arnold was an iconoclast. He was raised in an intellectually curious home in Guilford, Connecticut, by a mother who was a high school teacher, and a father who taught industrial engineering and dabbled in Democratic politics. One of Arnold's earliest political memories was having his father serve steamers to Bill Clinton, then the new governor of Arkansas, as he swung through town to campaign for a local politician.

Arnold's fascination with physiology began at the age of 11, when his grandfather gave him a set of weights and he started pumping iron in the garage. His first shot of steroids came after troubles with attention deficit disorder led him to drop out of the University of New Haven to work construction. The 10 pounds of muscle that he put on was such a revelation that, newly focused, he went back to school to earn a bachelor's degree in chemistry and a personal PhD in performance enhancement.

While floating through a series of ill-suited jobs (including a stint making hair-care products in New Jersey), Arnold became a regular on the cult Internet newsgroup *misc.fitness.weights.* The site, a virtual playground for wannabe gurus eager to boast about their breakthroughs, burst with enthusiasm for and news about performance-enhancing products. The speed with which theories were floated and then shot down was often dizzying. Dan Duchaine, of course, was revered by the group. But Arnold was starting to draw enough attention that one poster recently wrote, "Who is Patrick Arnold? I've never heard of him, but he sounds [*sic*] to know what the hells [*sic*] going on."

Duchaine reached the same conclusion. In e-mail exchanges, he encouraged Arnold just enough that the young chemist began sharing his ideas with the older man. Seeing those theories end up in The Guru's columns flattered Arnold, who finally got his chance to break into the industry when Duchaine recommended him to Bill Phillips at EAS. He went there at the beginning of the summer with high hopes, but his job as the company's research director turned out to be short-lived. Asked why in an interview years later, Arnold would say, "Bill was surrounded by old friends and I could tell I'd never be able to have my own identity there. Plus, I have an attention deficit problem. If I'm not excited, I can't do a good job."

By June, Arnold was back home in New Haven, hustling new ideas to make cash, when Duchaine told him about Antosh, who was hunting for a researcher to make his bold ideas about legal steroids a reality. Antosh had a partnership with a lab nestled in the farm country of Seymour, Illinois. He thought it would be a perfect place for Arnold to set up shop. Far from prying eyes, Arnold could do research on new applications of drugs while having access to a top-notch medical science library at the University of Illinois in nearby Champaign.

With the summer heat beating down, Arnold drove to Seymour in a 1986 Honda Civic, put himself up at a cheap hotel, and started hitting the books. Over the next six weeks, he turned up studies on 50 molecules and wrote summaries on each, sending them to Antosh in the Bay Area. Some looked promising but were ultimately rejected for practical reasons, either because they were too hard to obtain or had limited research done on them. But there was one that looked to Arnold like it could work, a compound called androstenedione.

A 1972 study from an obscure European journal revealed that androstenedione was just one molecular step away from testosterone. Antosh placed an order with a Chinese distribution company based in New Jersey for a small amount and told Arnold to mix it into capsules when it arrived. Then they would run a test to see if it worked.

GOLDEN, COLORADO
August 31, 1996

After sending the inflammatory kiss-off letter to his partners, Bill Phillips began to negotiate the buyout of EAS in earnest. He had agreed to give each of his partners five years of lucrative consulting fees in exchange for their 60 percent of the company. As they saw it, the deal was the best they could do under the circumstances; if they refused, Phillips would take his masterful marketing skills with him and they would likely be back to where they had started. For his part, Phillips couldn't wait to stamp EAS permanently with his super-sized ego. As soon as the deal closed, he set about building a new corporate monument to himself—a gleaming $6 million headquarters for EAS that was, in effect, the house that creatine built.

To christen it along with his growing celebrity, Phillips decided to throw a party on August 31. Duchaine arrived with his friend John Romano early in the evening, dressed in black tie. A red Lamborghini with a "ZOOOOM" license plate greeted them in the parking lot, as did a silver helicopter that had been waiting to shuttle VIP guests. Duchaine tried not to seem impressed, but Romano couldn't help himself. A few weeks earlier, Phillips had sent a first-class ticket to Romano in San Diego so he could make a personal pitch for Duchaine's protégé to work at *Muscle Media*. As the two men sat down in a lavishly appointed conference room, Phillips noticed that his guest had broken his expensive watch on the trip. With great fanfare, he summoned a smartly-tailored butler to have it fixed, ASAP.

Phillips was a master of the grand gesture, Romano thought. And as the chopper landed, he could see that the man was a good master of ceremonies, too. A red carpet and spotlights led them into a tent where ice sculptures dripped with champagne and *Playboy*-quality waitresses sauntered past with overflowing food trays. Phillips tried to add a dose of glamour to the Colorado night by inviting

Demi Moore, Sylvester Stallone, and even Arnold Schwarzenegger, creating a true VIP section should they arrive. None of them did, of course, so the friends made themselves comfortable, drinking expensive port and smoking cigars.

Watching Phillips work the room reminded Duchaine of how different the two men were, and why after everything he had been through, he was still basically living hand to mouth. Duchaine delighted in surprising people with his bluntness and caustic wit. Phillips, on the other hand, used his considerable charm. Writ large, that charisma allowed him to sell a simple product like creatine to tens of millions of customers. It was also clear that Phillips couldn't leave that part of his life behind fast enough.

As the night continued, Duchaine felt like the lone survivor of a bygone era, and he grew angrier and angrier about what he was seeing. Who were these pasty-faced people with their big stomachs and frozen faces, gorging themselves on the profits of an industry he had helped create? This wasn't what he had meant to start with the *Underground Steroid Handbook*. It made him sick inside. Sicker than he already was.

"Come on," he told Romano, suddenly upset with himself for coming at all. "Let's get the hell out of here."

The two had taken the helicopter back to the parking lot, when they heard Phillips take the stage to deliver some words. His soft voice carried over the PA system as he thanked his parents, his friends, and all the people who had come. "But there's one person I have to thank, above all," he said. "And that's Dan Duchaine."

"Shit," Duchaine muttered under his breath. "I guess we have to go back."

Romano watched from the back of the tent as his friend was called on stage to a huge round of applause. He had to hand it to Phillips—the man was the master of the grand gesture.

11

'CAUSE I'M TNT, I'M DYNAMITE!

November 28, 1996 - October 16, 1998

LAUSANNE, SWITZERLAND

November 28, 1996

Now that his lab at UCLA had become one of the largest Olympic drug-testing facilities in the world, Don Catlin was trying to keep a low profile. He had 16,000 samples coming through his doors annually, half from the Olympics and the rest from the NFL and NCAA. That kept him plenty busy without having to seek the limelight.

So when the International Olympic Committee asked Catlin to supervise steroid testing at the 1996 Atlanta Games, he accepted the task warily. He still hadn't forgotten the murky episode of the missing codes in Los Angeles 12 years earlier—the last time the Olympics had been held on American soil. The incident had ensured that half a dozen guilty athletes had gone home unpunished. Catlin worked too hard to catch cheaters to allow that to happen again. That's why he had arrived in Atlanta with a staff of 30 and several state-of-the-art machines. As he would say many years later, "You train three years for three weeks, and you have no idea what's about to come at you."

With more than 1,800 samples to analyze during the course of the Games, Catlin and his staff would have been on edge in the best of circumstances. But during the opening ceremonies, where the torch was lit by Muhammad Ali, he felt especially uncomfortable. Part of the unease had to do with the details no one had thought about beforehand, like accommodations. His staff was warehoused on the edge of town in a Motel 6 where they found drunks sleeping in the hallways. A young aide had clutched her bedsheets on the first night because she heard gunfire outside. But the real problem was the setup of the lab itself. It was housed inside a larger drug-testing operation run by the British pharmaceutical company SmithKline. Catlin had to beg every time he wanted to get a sample to run through a powerful new machine he had brought, an isotope ratio mass spectrometer that searched for below-normal amounts of Carbon-13 as a way of identifying excess testosterone. "Later," he was told. It was always later. The samples never arrived.

And then there was the dark cloud that literally hung over Atlanta on the evening of July 27. Catlin was working in the lab, studying stacks of readouts, when he saw workers racing for the doors. He grabbed one to ask, "What's happening?"

"It's the Olympic Village. A bomb just went off."

The terrorist explosion had killed a spectator and injured 111 others, further fraying the nerves of his already-exhausted staff. By the closing ceremonies, they had confirmed just two cases of steroid use—one by a Bulgarian triple jumper and another by a Russian hurdler. Yet Catlin's desk held five other files that concerned him. They were from athletes whose A-samples had tested positive. According to the rules, the doctor had to wait for a request from his Olympic superiors before he could proceed to confirm them by testing the matching B-sample.

As it happened, the same person whose request he awaited was the one who had discovered the loss of the fateful codes in Los Angeles—the IOC's medical czar, Prince Alexandre de Mérode of Belgium. Catlin waited and waited for de Mérode to give him the order. But, like the samples he sought, it never came.

Catlin's frustration mounted until he finally couldn't contain it. In a story that was published on November 17, Catlin told a reporter from the *Sunday Times* of London, "There were several other steroid positives from around the end of the Games which we reported. I can think of no reason why they have not been announced."

Once the story appeared, Catlin knew the Prince would read it as an attack. And now they were coming face-to-face for the first time since its publication at a Lausanne hotel where de Mérode was leading a meeting of the IOC's subcommittee on doping and biochemistry. Catlin wondered what the punishment would be for his candor. After all, people had been fired from the IOC for less. Well, Catlin figured, if it was his turn, at least he would be going out for the right reasons.

But de Mérode surprised him.

"Don, I see you've been busy," he said with a reproachful grin. When Catlin admitted he had, the Prince sighed. "Well now we must deal with it."

At the meeting attended by a half-dozen subcommittee members, de Mérode announced that he had serious reservations about the machine that was responsible for the five positives that Catlin had disclosed, a high-resolution mass spectrometer. It was too new to be trusted, he said.

Catlin bit his tongue. The Prince had been the one who approved the machines in the first place. What he was saying now was plainly just an excuse. It also showed the way things worked. He was dealing with it by burying the whole episode.

The Prince had once again decided that guilty athletes didn't need to be punished in his Olympic realm.

Stan Antosh was certain he was onto something with his new compound, androstenedione. While it wasn't as powerful as any of the steroids on the government's controlled substances list, its effect was measurable. Antosh discovered as much during his workouts. With his trial nearing, he had been hitting the weight room hard, trying to get himself into prison shape just in case things didn't break his way. Andro, he found, helped him recover faster and work out longer. Of course, there were some side effects, like soreness in his breast area. But he didn't have it as bad as the guys in the gyms who were quadrupling his recommendation and taking eight capsules a day. Besides, the consensus was that it was a tolerable price to pay for a legal steroid precursor.

Working out of a small office above a friend's vitamin store, Antosh ordered five kilograms of androstenedione powder from his Chinese connection and sold out the first batch within two weeks of its arrival. It seemed that every trainer in the Bay Area's gyms was hoarding the stuff, and most had a professional athlete or two among their clients. One of the stars who had heard about Andro was the Giants' left fielder, Barry Bonds. The 32-year-old All-Star got Antosh's number through a friend on the San Francisco 49ers and called early one evening to say, "I'm losing bat speed. What do you have that can help me?"

The next day, Antosh walked around his friend's vitamin store, picking out things that he thought would be good for Bonds. Scanning one shelf, he grabbed a bottle called Rock of Ages, which was made from juniper berries that had been scraped off rocks in the Himalayas. On another, he spied Build Up, liver pills made from the liquefied organs of cattle raised in Argentina. He tossed in some methylsulfonylmethane, which he thought would help ease Bonds's joint pain. And he added a bit of tyrosine, an amino acid from cheese that converted to noradrenaline in the body for an energy boost.

A few months later, Antosh recommended Androstene 50. Like creatine, it wasn't the strongest thing to hit baseball's clubhouses, but it was helping push everyday players to explore their physiological limits and reach the divide that McGwire, Canseco, and Giambi, among others, had already crossed.

CARLSBAD, CALIFORNIA

March 1997

The one time that Dan Duchaine met Don Catlin occurred in the mid-1980s, when Catlin occupied a cramped office on the UCLA campus and Duchaine called to ask if they could get together. Duchaine was just nosing around, trying to figure out what Catlin knew. After an hour, he hadn't learned much, but he still thanked the doctor for his time and left.

Since then, Duchaine hadn't thought much about Catlin, mainly because he worked in bodybuilding, a sport where Catlin had no real influence. But things were starting to come full circle, thanks to a new company Duchaine had set up to cash in on his reputation: Guru, Inc.

For $350 an hour, Duchaine offered callers advice on how to get the body of their dreams. Pro wrestlers got tips on growing cartoon muscles. Hollywood action stars were told how to become chiseled for the cameras. Even cops called, looking for an edge. Duchaine didn't care. He was democratic about whose money he took.

According to his then-business manager, Laura Moore, one early Guru, Inc. customer was Bill Romanowski of the Denver Broncos. (Romanowski says he has no recollection of ever speaking to Duchaine or calling the helpline.) The linebacker who was on his way to a record 243 consecutive games already had quite the professional entourage: five chiropractors, four acupuncturists, three nutritionists, two massage therapists, one speed coach, and one trainer. But there was always room for another Guru. Over time, Moore watched Duchaine's name spread to roughly 50 players. Even strength coaches got into the act. So many callers had the same question—tell me about human growth hormone and insulin—that Duchaine typed out instructions for Moore to read to clients so he wouldn't even have to get on the phone.

Another service of Guru, Inc. was a newsletter that Duchaine was launching called *Dirty Dieting: Militant Muscle Growth and Fast Fat Loss*. Its first cover story, "The Poor Man's Guide to Making GHB," revealed everything about the different directions he and Bill Phillips were traveling in.

"Now that GHB has gained notoriety in the news media," it read, "purchasing the necessary chemicals will become more difficult to do, so some subterfuge may be required." It advised readers to get the main ingredient, gamma-butyrolactone (which could be found in paint remover), from one supply store and to go to another for the second, the active agent in Drano. One can only imagine the types of people who followed the advice, and what happened to them—or those they intoxicated—as a result.

Elsewhere, he pushed things just as far. There was "Dan's Deviant Delights," a column in which he followed the exploits of friends from the bodybuilding world who were making side money filming gay porn. And there were forums in which he gave his chemical friends free rein. The debut issue contained a column by Patrick Arnold, who described the complicated process of synthesizing a steroid called methyltrienolone. (In a few years, Arnold would build on that knowledge to create a designer steroid that would become infamous.) In sum, the publication was meant to show Duchaine's rebel underground—or at least what was left of it—and that its leader hadn't lost his edge.

But in private, Duchaine was feeling increasingly trapped by the image he had created for himself. What was it that he had said to his old friend, Mike Zumpano, those many years ago? "I may be going to prison. But you're the one already in prison, with your little life." Apparently, there were all sorts of prisons. And after serving two terms in the federal kind, he was just now realizing that The Guru character he had created for himself had become one all its own.

Now 44, the alarm on Duchaine's biological clock had gone off and he was obsessed with having a family. He told friends that he desperately wanted a son and was trying to keep in shape so he could raise one. He took long rides along the coast, looking stylish in spandex shorts and a sleeveless shirt as he peddled his low-slung, recumbent bike.

But he was still no closer to finding Ms. Right. His latest relationship involved a newlywed from Ohio who was wading in the world of competitive bodybuilding as a way to fill empty hours while her husband finished law school. She had sought Duchaine out on *misc.fitness.weights,* and after a few pleasant exchanges, he e-mailed her to say that he was planning a trip to the East Coast. Would she like to meet?

Her name was Mary Lou[1] and on a sweltering day in August 1996, she set out to meet him on Long Island, New York. The purpose of the trip was to have another plastic surgery procedure to add hair plugs to his scalp. When Mary Lou found him in his hotel room, he was drinking a beer, with his head still bandaged and tubes draining excess blood.

"Have a drink," he offered. She had one, then three, and began to open up about her ambitions. Out of nowhere, Duchaine applied a tourniquet to begin injecting himself with Nubain. When he handed her a syringe, Mary Lou tried to seem nonchalant. "This is the stuff you need," he said, watching her inch away. "It'll help you train through the pain."

She had never done much more than smoke a joint, but Mary Lou agreed, and in that one moment, her life became forever

---

1 Her name and some identifying details have been changed.

changed. The next morning, Duchaine was still sleeping when she awoke and decided to get them breakfast. While Mary Lou was waiting at a diner, her stomach seized up on her and her insides burned. She returned to the hotel room shaking. "What's happening to me?" she asked.

"You need another hit," he said. She took it, gratefully, and after some more sex, was given a small bottle of Nubain to take back home with her.

Throughout the fall, Duchaine kept sending Mary Lou plain brown packages by mail, hooking her more and more deeply. When a package didn't come in mid-October, she called in a panic and he suggested that to get more, she meet him for the weekend in Maine, where he would be visiting his aunt. To outsiders, they probably looked like the typical kind of lovers who come to New England in the autumn. Except they were higher than hell the whole time.

By March 1997, Mary Lou had all but completed the journey from bored housewife to Nubain junkie. As his former lovers had discovered, Duchaine could be very warm when he wanted, but he could also be cruel. While they were lying in bed on one of their Nubain getaways, he told Mary Lou, "You know what I hate about you? Your skin." He felt it was too loose for competitive bodybuilding, especially the upcoming nationals in Dallas. She needed to get the translucent, shrink-wrapped look that judges liked. As it happened, he had just the ticket: an industrial chemical named Dinitrophenol.

DNP, as it is known, was employed in the early 1900s to ignite explosives. But German researchers found that it led to drastic weight loss when swallowed because it caused the body to burn calories as heat instead of storing them as fat. By turning the internal thermostat way up, DNP, which is similar in structure to TNT, can increase one's metabolism by as much as 50 percent. It is literally like playing with fire and users can incinerate their insides if they take too much.

The key to DNP is knowing how much to take. When he first got his hands on a sample of the yellow powder, Duchaine asked John Romano to help him put it into gel capsules. After a while, Romano couldn't understand why he felt so hot. Finally, it occurred to him that the two of them were absorbing the powder through their pores. His temperature had soared to 103 degrees.

Mary Lou was a willing subject, perhaps too willing. One day she took more DNP than Duchaine had advised and started burning up. Unable to reach Duchaine, she called his aide, Bruce Kneller, to ask what was happening to her. "How much are you taking?" he asked. When she told him, he was aghast. "If you keep that up, you're going to die." Duchaine hit the roof when he heard that Kneller had advised his girlfriend without his permission.

"Stay out of my business," he yelled over the phone. "Better still, stay out of my life."

LOS ANGELES
October 1997

Don Catlin was irritated by Andro. It was one thing to find a new steroid that someone like Dan Duchaine was trying to slip past him. There was a certain frisson from outwitting someone who was trying to outwit you. But from where Catlin sat in his Los Angeles lab, there was nothing chemically challenging about Andro. It was a one-trick pony: You swallowed it and it metabolized into testosterone. That's why they called it a steroid precursor.

Actually, Andro was just the beginning. In the past several months, a slew of copycats had come tumbling out of the supplement industry. Osmo introduced a stronger version of Andro named 4-AD and a company called Mass Quantities was selling pills that metabolized into the long-lasting steroid Nandrolone. Catlin had an over-the-counter steroid avalanche on his hands. If that wasn't bad enough, he was also on the business end of mislabeled or contaminated supplements that were causing banned substances to show up in unsuspecting athletes' urine samples.

What bothered him was all the extra work it created for his overtaxed staff. Every positive test required them to confirm and reconfirm his work, and for him to testify about it in disciplinary hearings. All this for what Catlin considered a junk supplement that was unlikely to enhance performance.

The most troubling part of it was how all of this was distracting him from the real work that needed to be done. Human growth hormone was supposedly so prevalent in Atlanta, the Olympics were being called the HGH Games. A test for it was desperately needed.

If Senator Orrin Hatch wanted to slow down the doping fight, he couldn't have done better than pushing a bill like DSHEA.

SAN DIEGO

January 25, 1998

Bill Romanowski opened up the tackle box he had brought with him to Qualcomm Stadium and proudly showed it off to the reporters gathered around him. Divided into neat sections were 500 pills that amounted to a tasting menu from the kitchen of the NFL's most lunatic linebacker. If there was an heir to Lyle Alzado, it was Romo.

Just five weeks earlier, he had been forced to apologize for spitting in the face of a 49ers wide receiver on *Monday Night Football* after a play was whistled dead. Though no one would ever accuse the two-time Super Bowl winner of letting intellect overshadow his instincts—the *San Francisco Chronicle*'s Tim Keown once wrote that if not for football, Romo would "be sitting on the steps of a trailer somewhere, whittling away and trying to figure out how his overalls got stuck in that tree"—Romanowski was a student of how to both endure and inflict pain, and had done plenty of both to reach Super Bowl XXXII against the Green Bay Packers.

Romanowski was also shrewd about playing the press. As soon as he learned that Bill Phillips had signed tight end Shannon Sharpe as a spokesman for EAS, he told Phillips that he could generate twice the publicity for half the money. And damned if he wasn't as good as his word. Before the first down of Super Bowl XXXII had been played, Romanowski had helped Phillips score the coup of his career. A television audience of 133 million fans watched not just Romo and Sharpe, but running back Terrell Davis and quarterback John Elway giving interviews in EAS gear.

The game itself was a public relations dream. The undersized Broncos held off the driving Packers in the fourth quarter to win 31-24 and the theme of the next day's stories was that the team's superior conditioning had sealed the win. As *The Seattle Times* noted, Gilbert Brown, Green Bay's 345-pound defensive tackle, was so tired he could barely pull himself off the field after plays. "They're winded! They're winded!" the Broncos kept yelling from the sideline. Mark Schlereth, a Denver offensive guard, boasted to the *Baltimore Sun*, "We had them on their heels the entire game. Heck, I wasn't even tired."

Phillips's public relations bonanza left executives at the NFL's offices in New York dumbfounded. There would be a lot of finger-pointing about existing licensing deals, and how EAS had managed to circumvent them without paying the league. The NFL also announced it would start levying fines for anyone who wore unapproved gear.

But it was too late. Anyone who watched the Super Bowl in San Diego got the message that Romo's tackle box had helped to work a miracle. It would take months for evidence to emerge that Romanowski was also on steroids and human growth hormone. But by then Phillips would have sold his stake in EAS for tens of millions, once again having shrewdly figured how to cash out when his hand was the hottest.

The morning was just coming into focus for Willy Voet as he raced down the E17 motorway toward the French border.

Voet was the *soigneur*, or physical therapist, for France's top cycling team, Festina. But the true nature of his job was reflected in the ice coolers behind his front seat. Inside lay 24 vials of human growth hormone and testosterone, 234 doses of the endurance booster erythropoietin (EPO), and 60 capsules of a blood thinner called Asaflow, which balanced the blood-thickening effects of EPO. In all, it was enough to prepare his team for the Tour de France, which was due to start in Dublin later that week.

When Voet set out from his apartment in Veynes, France, the day before, he had taken the drugs from the vegetable bin of his refrigerator and loaded them into the coolers in his family car. Then he had set off for Paris, where he moved everything into the Festina team car that he was now driving, and headed 180 miles away to Ghent to get more EPO from the team's doctor. Twelve hours later, he finally called it a night at a friend's apartment in Brussels.

Having just celebrated his 53rd birthday, Voet felt every bit of his age when he got up at 5:30 a.m. to continue his journey. To fortify himself for the three-hour drive to Calais and the ferry to England, he injected himself with a potent mixture called a Belgian cocktail— a high-octane mix of heroin, cocaine, caffeine, and amphetamines. As he buzzed along the motorway, Voet felt as if he could drive for another two days straight.

With France finally in sight, Voet remembered a warning that the team doctor gave him—be careful of border police. At the last second, he turned his wheel to the right, guiding the gaudily colored pace car down a side road populated by farmhouses. At 6:45 a.m. on a typical Wednesday, Voet figured he would be able to pass through unnoticed. He immediately realized the error of that judgment when he saw a customs officer laying in wait on the roadside.

As he would go on to write in his memoir, *Breaking the Chain*, Voet didn't think about the banned drugs in the cooler behind his seat as he slowed to a halt, at least not at first. He was more concerned about the two full vials of Belgian cocktail in the knapsack beside him. Maybe the *gendarme* was just a cycling fan, attracted by the Festina name on the car, he thought. Then he caught sight of a white van with four other agents hiding in the bushes. No, he soon realized, this wasn't about autographs.

Before the first officer reached his window, Voet slipped a hand inside the knapsack, grabbed one of the vials and slid it into his trousers. The other was still in his hand when the officer asked, "Anything to declare?"

"Just vitamins for the riders," he said.

When the officer motioned him to get out, Voet casually flicked the other vial into the woods. The officer seemed not to notice. Maybe he had dodged a bullet after all, he thought.

In fact, Voet was about to become front-page news around the world. "What are these?" the lead agent asked, pulling back the front seat to reveal the coolers that Voet had so carefully packed with sealed Tupperware containers.

Voet shrugged. "Stuff to help the riders recover, I think."

The agent instructed Voet to drive to the customs office a few miles away. The *soigneur* managed to move the vial that he had hidden in his trousers into his underwear, but that was discovered during a subsequent strip search. The drugs that were supposed to be crossing the channel with him were immediately sent off to a lab to be analyzed. After being X-rayed for drugs that the agents suspected he was carrying inside his body (he wasn't), Voet was placed in a holding cell for the night.

The next day, he awoke exhausted. Besides having had two nights with next to no sleep, he had come down from his heroin-and-coke high in a cement cell that smelled like hot puke. Still, Voet might have maintained his composure if he hadn't overheard a TV news report in which Festina's riders were selling him out, insisting that all the drugs belonged to Voet and not them.

Feeling desperately alone and forsaken, Voet broke. Over the next week, he told the agents everything they wanted to know about the Tour de France's secrets. He acknowledged that he was the courier for drugs that his team's doctor had administered, and that its director financed the buys through a connection in Portugal. His wife also handed over books that Festina officials encouraged her to burn—books that showed the doping program was a team affair and not the work of some rogue *soigneur*. (Voet was eventually given a 10-month suspended sentence and fined for his involvement; the team director was given a one-year suspended sentence and fined for administering, aiding, and abetting the using of doping substances and procedures during a sports competition; the team doctor was charged with importing and illegal transport of poisonous substances, and was awaiting trial in Belgium when he died of cancer.)

Europe's dailies hung on every new development. "Police Question Festina Officials," *The Independent* of London reported on July 16. A day later, *The Guardian* noted, "Festina boss suspended but team claims 'clear conscience.'" Technically, the Festina affair wasn't an Olympic problem. Though cycling was an Olympic sport, the Tour de France handled its own testing. Nevertheless, this was happening in the IOC's backyard so it demanded *some* response.

On July 26—nearly a decade to the day that the Ben Johnson scandal erupted—Olympic leader Juan Samaranch stepped forward. The Spanish aristocrat didn't spend a lot of time thinking about doping. His job involved silencing scandal, not inviting it. Yet the political miscalculation of his remark was still breathtaking.

In a conversation with a reporter for the Spanish daily *El Mundo*, Samaranch confided that he had two issues with doping. The first, he said, is that it is "harmful to an athlete's health." The second is that "it artificially augments his performance." Had he stopped there, he would have been fine. But the aging Samaranch went on to draw a distinction only a businessman could love: "If it's just the second case," he added, then "for me that's not doping."

Reading the remark in his lab in Los Angeles, Don Catlin buried his head in his hands. The cycling scandal involving Willy Voet proved what he had been saying all along: that things were getting worse, not better. EPO? Asaflow? They made Ben Johnson's stanozonol look quaint by comparison.

Yet the best the leader of the Olympic movement could do was to say he didn't think any of it was wrong.

LOMPOC, CALIFORNIA
August 23, 1998

Stan Antosh still had the smell of manure in his nose as he rode the prison van back from his morning shift at work. He had been incarcerated since March, thanks to a trial that left him convicted of failure to register a drug manufacturing facility in the early 1990s. The Bureau of Prisons had assigned him to a minimum-security camp in Lompoc, California, and fortunately for the one-time farm boy, it had a dairy. He volunteered to serve his time by waking up at 3 a.m. to wash cow manure out of the stalls.

This particular morning was uneventful, and he was planning on taking a nap after the shift ended. But no sooner had he returned to his dorm than an inmate greeted him by pointing to a TV in the corner. "Hey, Antosh," he said. "Check out ESPN. You're a star."

The network, which had been actively covering Mark McGwire's pursuit of Roger Maris's single-season home run record, was reporting a story about Andro being found in the Cardinals' locker room. Antosh turned up the volume. An Associated Press reporter had seen it firsthand and was causing controversy by reporting that it was banned by the NFL and NCAA, but not by Major League

Baseball. Antosh searched for a copy of the day's paper so he could read the story himself. It started: "Sitting on the top shelf of Mark McGwire's locker, next to a can of Popeye spinach and packs of sugarless gum, is a brown bottle labeled Androstenedione."

Antosh's whole body tingled. He knew that McGwire used Andro because the St. Louis first baseman endorsed Champion Nutrition and Antosh sold his excess supply to its owner, Mike Zumpano. "That's my Andro," he thought.

He asked permission to use the prison phone and immediately called his girlfriend, who was running Osmo in his absence. "Oh my God, Stan," she said, relieved to hear from him. "The phone's been ringing off the hook. We have 800 kilos in stock and it's all going be sold by the end of the week."

Antosh hung up the phone and returned to his prison bunk, too wired for a nap. He did some quick calculations in his head. If his girlfriend was right, he was going to make $68,000 this week.

"I'll be damned," he thought. Thanks to Mark McGwire, he was having the richest single week of his life. And it was happening while he was in prison.

TIJUANA, MEXICO
October 16, 1998

Whether Dan Duchaine loved Mary Lou was irrelevant. He probably did, in his own way. But he wanted a child so much that he would tell her anything. On a visit to Scottsdale, Arizona, he walked into a jewelry store and walked out with a two-and-a-half carat diamond ring. At dinner that night, he slid it across the table and said, "I want to marry you. I want us to make a baby."

But even through her Nubain haze, Mary Lou had difficulty saying yes. She was still trying to hang onto the shards of her pre-Dan life, and she wasn't far enough gone to make herself his junkie bride. At least, not yet.

Mary Lou had lost everything—her husband, her friends, her life back East. For a time, all that she had left was her bodybuilding dream. And Duchaine had ruined that as well. She was clearly worse off than when she had first visited him in that Long Island hotel room two years earlier. The DNP he had given her caused her skin to look sickly yellow and Nubain made her lethargic. As for competitive bodybuilding, she had gotten knocked out of the 1997 Nationals in Dallas in the first round, and with the 1998 show a month away, Mary Lou could see the same thing as everyone else: she looked like hell.

Duchaine's solution was another one of his short cuts: "You need calf implants." Calf implants? Well, she thought, it's not any crazier than taking TNT.

All of which explained why they had set out this morning from Carlsbad to a clinic located half an hour over the border in Mexico. Duchaine checked her into the clinic, then got a hotel room and came back just as she was being wheeled into surgery. "You'll be fine," he said.

The operation was done in the late afternoon and quickly declared a success. Mary Lou was given some sedatives and told to rest. In fact, it hadn't gone well. Not at all. Mary Lou realized as much when she awoke in the middle of the night with her feet incredibly numb. It felt, she would later remember, like a terrible case of frostbite. She dragged herself to the nurse's station, but the nurse didn't speak English and ordered her back to bed. The next morning, she awoke to see the result. Because the blood vessels in her legs had not been properly re-attached during the prior day's surgery, her lower body was essentially cut off from her circulatory system. She was rushed into the operating room so the implants, now leaking silicone, could be removed. Seeing her leg sliced open on either side as though it had zippers made Mary Lou grow faint. But before she passed out, she screamed, "I want to go to an American hospital!"

An ambulance raced her back across the border with Duchaine following closely behind. By the time they pulled up to the emergency room of Scripps Mercy Hospital in San Diego, Mary Lou's kidneys and liver were in a state of near-failure, leaving her dangerously close to death.

Disaster didn't begin to describe the next 30 days. She was in a constant state of agony as surgeons tried to stabilize her with one operation after another. Finally, as she started coming around, the medical staff gave her the grim prognosis.

Dan Duchaine's third wife, Shelley Harvey, was in England, trying to recover from the brain damage he had caused. Now the woman he wanted to replace her, a woman whom he had promised prize-winning legs, was about to have one of them sawed off.

12

THE KING IS DEAD

February 4, 1999 - January 13, 2000

If there was any doubt about the power the head of the Olympic movement could wield, Juan Antonio Samaranch was demonstrating it in Lausanne. With a stroke of his pen, he had ordered 600 delegates from the IOC and ministers from the world's governments to a first-of-its-kind summit on drugs in sport. Samaranch may not have understood doping, but he clearly comprehended the way his remarks about Festina had weakened him at the moment he could afford it least. The IOC was being swallowed whole by a bribery scandal in which five members had already resigned for taking cash to help Salt Lake City land the 2002 Winter Games. He needed to appear tough on corruption.

The idea for the summit had been hatched well before the Salt Lake bribery allegations surfaced. In August 1998, Samaranch ordered his top aide, Canadian attorney Dick Pound, to focus on the drug issue. Pound proposed creating a single drug-testing agency that would oversee all Olympic sports. As revolutionary as the idea might have seemed, Samaranch saw its practical advantages. An anti-doping agency could standardize the list of banned drugs and the punishments for using them. It was also going to be expensive; Pound put its initial budget at $25 million. But they would ask the world's governments for help at the summit. What Samaranch didn't want was a stranger running this important and empowered agency. Days before the summit was to start, he announced that he wanted to oversee it personally. His longtime medical advisor, Prince Alexandre de Mérode of Belgium, would handle the day-to-day affairs.

Arriving in Switzerland, Don Catlin felt rebelliousness in the air. He had no real problems with Samaranch and, despite their run-ins, respected the Prince. But the Salt Lake scandal had galvanized the opposition to both men. Summing up the dissatisfied mood, Germany's interior minister, Otto Schily, told reporters: "Everyone must know when it's time to go."

To Catlin, the most impressive member of the American delegation was Barry McCaffrey, the retired general representing the Clinton Administration as its drug czar. A Vietnam veteran, McCaffrey served in the Gulf War and oversaw United States forces in Central and South America before going to work for the White House. Unlike the Olympic regulars who usually spoke for America, McCaffrey was a tornado of a presence—a man who knew exactly what he wanted.

McCaffrey was troubled by Mark McGwire's use of Andro and the repercussions it was having on America's youth. The St. Louis slugger was now an icon for hitting 70 home runs in the 1998 season, finally breaking Roger Maris's record of 61, and giving the country one of the feel-good moments of the year. As a result, Andro sales among kids had skyrocketed five-fold. A study in the journal *Pediatrics* found that an alarming 2.7 percent of Massachusetts's middle-school athletes were using actual steroids.

McCaffrey supported the idea of an anti-doping agency that could patrol the borders of sport. Even if it only had power over the Olympics, it could draw important lines and establish definitions for cheating. But he wasn't going to use American dollars to fund another one of Samaranch's pet projects.

When Samaranch gaveled the session to order on February 2, it was clear how little stomach the 78-year-old had for the subject. "We are not a court," he explained, "and do not wish to become one." Perhaps not, but when it was McCaffrey's time to address the assembly, he was determined to put the Olympic chief on trial. "Lack of accountability and failure of leadership have challenged the legitimacy of this institution," the general boomed. "The IOC must operate as a democratic and accountable public institution."

With that, it was war. Jacques Rogge, the suave Belgian who ran the executive committee, used Mark McGwire to attack McCaffrey, showing what a political problem the slugger was becoming for America. "If you go on [with a] moralizing and lecturing tone, you must be sure your own house is in order," he said.

And so it went over three hectic days. To Catlin, the loneliest figure at the summit was de Mérode. Whatever else could be said of him, the Prince was a proud man, yet he was watching his power base crumble. He hadn't helped himself earlier in the week by suggesting that the best way to fight doping was to reduce penalties. (He argued that the shorter penalties wouldn't be challenged as quickly in court.) But de Mérode wasn't going to let himself be ridiculed, either. In an astonishing reversal, he stunned reporters by blaming Samaranch for the mess they were in. Claiming that he had had the idea for an anti-doping agency 10 years earlier, the Prince told the French newspaper *L'Equipe*, "Samaranch was opposed. The plan was shot down by 90 percent of the people who today are in favor [of it]." But the Prince's ultimate undoing was his own imperious nature. In what many considered the signature moment of hubris at the summit, he waved off a breakthrough blood test for HGH that had been developed by a leading British endocrinologist. De Mérode was openly contemptuous of it, refusing to let the doctor speak at an Olympic press conference and saying it needed millions more dollars of work.

By Thursday, Samaranch was eager to declare any kind of victory that he could and return home before more damage was done. Having withdrawn his clumsy idea to head the doping agency, he threw the question of leadership to a working group. He also capitulated to the soccer and cycling officials who had balked at the idea of a mandatory two-year ban for first-time offenders. (A provision was inserted allowing reviews for "exceptional circumstances.") What was left was a six-point "declaration" that pledged to field a working anti-doping agency for the Sydney Olympics in 2000. Putting on a brave face, Samaranch leaned formally into the microphone and told the delegates: "I ask you to adopt this declaration. Agree?"

A *Los Angeles Times* reporter described what happened next: "A ripple of mild applause followed. No show of hands, just a low-level clapping with many members of the audience abstaining. Samaranch did not ask if anyone disagreed. Flashing a self-satisfied grin, he quickly clacked his gavel and pronounced the declaration passed."

Catlin left the summit feeling exhausted but hopeful. After spending 15 years feeling like his work was on the Olympic back burner, the world had come together to put it front and center, and the Sydney Olympics would be the first to be monitored by this new police force.

CARLSBAD, CALIFORNIA
Spring 1999

After her amputation, Mary Lou spent a month living in Dan Duchaine's apartment, drugged out on OxyContin, morphine, and

Valium. But not Nubain. She had kicked that. And having done so, she began to see The Guru through different eyes. For the first time, she noticed how needlessly cruel he could be. "You know," he said one night, "you don't turn me on any more."

He couldn't even help her indulge the hope of walking on a prosthetic leg. "It'll never happen," Duchaine told her, brushing it aside like so much nonsense. "You're spending the rest of your life in a wheelchair." Burnt and broken, she called her estranged husband and begged him to take her back. By the new year, Mary Lou and Duchaine were living on separate coasts.

With his dream of fathering a child crushed, Duchaine looked around at what he had left. The steroid industry bored him. At 46, he had tried all there was to try, written about everything that interested him. It was clear now that there would be no revolution, at least not the kind he envisioned many years ago. He had been a rebel and a smuggler and a martyr, a prisoner and a writer and a lover. And what did it all get him? He was weak, balding, middle aged, and alone. He began to think about opening that bike store he had wanted when he first came to California. He also started to write one-act plays, trying to find that young theater student wedged deep inside of him.

For comfort, Duchaine reached out to a curvaceous blonde he had met two years earlier at The Arnold Expo in Ohio. "Big tits and an expert on steroids—my kind of girl," Duchaine told Shelley Hominuk, a model and fitness writer who frequently covered the subject, when they first met. Years later, she would insist that they were only friends, though he clearly wanted them to be more, and she helped him through his breakup with Mary Lou by taking him out to the theater and opera.

But by the spring of 1999, it was clear that a piece of Duchaine was irrevocably broken. When he sighed and said, "The things that matter most I don't get," it was hard not to sense that he was looking back on his life's work. Pat Arnold was the star of the underground now—young, brash, and an actual chemist. Though Arnold still consulted with him from time to time, that was just a courtesy. He didn't need The Guru anymore. Duchaine feared that no one did.

This realization caused a profound change to settle over him. In March, Mary Lou returned to California to see her doctors and crashed on his couch. Out of nowhere, he began crying like a baby, saying how much he loved her, how sorry he was that he had ruined her life. "I'd never seen that side of him before," she would say.

Soon thereafter, he called Hominuk sounding more scared than she had ever heard him. His blood pressure was rising and because he had no health insurance, he couldn't afford to stay in a hospital overnight. Could she come by to stay with him until morning? She said of course, and at dawn, she drove him to the ER. He came out looking awful.

Did he know that he was dying, that the cysts on his kidneys were like water-filled balloons, choking the life out of him? Probably. In the morning, he got up feeling as though he had partied hard the night before, when in fact he was going to bed earlier and earlier. The bathroom mirror showed a grey-haired man who looked like he could be a senior citizen. As the summer wore on, he began arranging his papers and his life. He wrote a living will and handed it to Hominuk.

"I'm not taking this," she said.

"You don't understand," he replied, pleadingly.

NEW YORK CITY
Fall 1999

A man who considers where he has been inevitably turns to the places he hasn't, and Dan Duchaine was thinking more and more about New York. Ever since his drama days in Boston, he dreamt about living in the city—gorging on its shows, museums, and restaurants. Sensing that he didn't have much longer, he rented an apartment on Manhattan's Upper East Side.

New York was everything Duchaine had imagined. To a stranger, he was just another old man shuffling down its busy streets. But as he disappeared into the city, he lived the life he once envisioned for himself. One day he had lunch at the newly renovated Russian Tea Room, and the next he was taking in a Broadway show.

But as winter settled over the city, he was hit with an intractable flu. His voice was hoarse most of the time and the tremble in his hand had become even more pronounced. Just before Christmas, Duchaine arranged to meet Mary Lou for dinner at Windows on the World atop the World Trade Center. It was a sad holiday meal between old lovers trying not to let hate into their hearts. With the city brilliantly illuminated below them, Dan told her, "I finally did what you said and went to a doctor."

"And what did he say?"

"He said I should go to a kidney specialist."

"Are you?"

"No." He was actually heading to Connecticut to see his sister for Christmas Eve, and then to Maine to visit his aunt before coming back to the city so he could usher in the year 2000 in Times Square. "Come with me," he said.

It was a last attempt to repair his life, to invest in the future. But looking at the shadow of a man she once admired, all Mary Lou could do was slide her hand out from under his.

"You're not attracted to me anymore?" he asked.

She looked down. "It's over between us, Dan."

On Christmas Eve, Duchaine piled himself in a rental car to be with his sister Sheila and her family. His appearance shocked her. He brought Christmas presents for the kids but it was hard to feel festive with the scent of sickness permeating his body. Sheila served a sumptuous ham for dinner, but he couldn't finish what was on his plate without falling asleep. After her husband and children tiptoed out of the room, she bent over her snoring brother.

"Dan, you really need to see someone."

"No, I don't," he muttered drowsily.

"You think you know more than doctors, don't you?"

"Uh huh."

When Sheila sent him off the next morning to spend Christmas Day in Maine, she was worried. His hacking cough swallowed his farewells and she asked if he wouldn't rather stay instead of making the four-hour drive north. He brushed off the suggestion, then waved goodbye.

By the time he got to his Aunt Loraine's home, he could barely stay awake. The house was decorated for the season, but he walked past the presents and tinsel, right to the room in the attic he had used as a child. Its walls were filled with photos of a simpler era: Dan smiling with his adoptive father. Dan acting in a high school play. Dan clowning outside his dorm at Boston University.

Dan fell asleep.

He never made it to Times Square. After a few days, he told his Aunt Loraine that he needed to get home as fast as he could. The newspapers were filled with stories about how air travel might be unsafe because of a glitch in computer software called the "Millennium Bug." Some sports teams had even grounded their players, fearing for their safety. But Duchaine took a flight that ensured he would be in the air when the famous ball dropped. He landed on the West Coast shortly after midnight Pacific time, while the entire country was toasting its next thousand years.

His first call was to Shelley Hominuk, who was surprised to hear from him. "Dan, what are you doing here?" she said, cupping her hand over her free ear to drown out the noise of a party going full blast.

"I'll explain later. Can you come get me at the airport?"

"I can't, Dan. I've got a house full of people. I'll call you tomorrow."

He put down the phone. It was starting to rain. He tried to find a taxi, but the stand was empty. He waited awhile in the rain, his cough getting worse and worse.

> ### CARLSBAD, CALIFORNIA
> *January 13, 2000*

Shelley Hominuk was in a post office near her home, mailing a letter, when an elderly man with a walker tripped right in front of her. As she helped him up, she thought of Duchaine. He called almost every day, but she hadn't heard from him since Monday. Something's wrong, she told herself. After trying to reach him all day, she headed to Carlsbad in a driving rainstorm to see what that might be.

Shortly before 10 p.m., Hominuk arrived to find the house quiet. The kit cars that Duchaine prized so much were sitting under canvas covers in his driveway. She felt the hoods. Cold.

Using a spare key he had given her, Hominuk let herself in. "Dan? *Dan?*"

The downstairs was quiet, so she made her way up a stairwell to the second floor, where his bedroom was. The door was ajar and she opened it slowly. At first, it looked to her like he was just sleeping. *"Dan?"*

As Hominuk drew closer, she could see that the yellow tinge of his skin had turned pale blue. She bent down and touched him. His chest, instead of rising and falling, was stiff. She took a deep breath and tried to calm herself. Looking around, she saw things she felt no one should find near a dead man, like his porn collection. She discreetly gathered it up and then called 911. A police cruiser arrived in minutes.

Considering how sick he had become in his last few months, Dan Duchaine's death should have caught no one off guard. And yet it did. His will stipulated that he wanted to be cremated and flown back to Maine, so Hominuk hastily arranged a ceremony in Carlsbad and invited a handful of people to join her. A second service held in Maine was better attended, but only because his aunt filled it with her friends from church. The obituary that ran in the January 16 edition of Maine's *Portland Press Herald* quoted her as saying, "People said he was a loner or an outlaw, but that didn't bother him."

That wasn't really true. Dan Duchaine had a deep need for kinship. His friend John Romano showed as much when he wrote in a tribute: "I still find myself—nearly daily—wondering ... what we'd be talking about today if he were alive ... and what he would have told me had I made it up to New York the last time he so vehemently implored me to visit."

Many of those who had walked in and out of his life found themselves wondering the same thing. When Duchaine entered Gold's Gym in Venice for the first time in 1980, he was an actor looking for a stage. What he stumbled into, at least in the beginning, was a crusade. He predicted a future in which people would use steroids to stay young and healthy forever. To him, steroids were America's Drug.

Along the way, the great crusader lost his faith. In the course of a ruinous drug odyssey, Duchaine stopped caring about health, or even being healthy. His two biological sisters had also contracted polycystic kidney disease, yet they both survived him, raising questions about whether the growth drugs he took might have exacerbated the cysts on his kidneys.

The greatest loss following Dan Duchaine's death wasn't to the friends who mourned him, or even the women who might have found a way to love him. It was to the revolution he started.

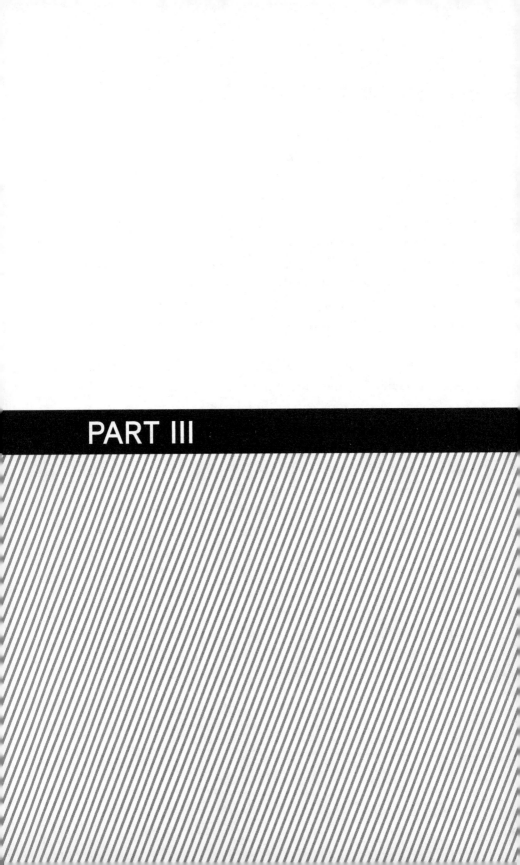

PART III

LONG LIVE THE KING

2000-PRESENT

13

THE RIGHT STUFF

February 25, 2000 - November 17, 2000

February 25, 2000

Arnold Schwarzenegger knew the clock was ticking on his action movie career. At 52, the Terminator was considerably thinner than just a few years ago. The difference was apparent while he was filming *The 6th Day* in Vancouver. After recent heart valve surgery, Schwarzenegger could no longer pretend he was the iron man of old. *The 6th Day* would gross a disappointing $34.6 million—a little more than a third of what his *Eraser* had taken in a few years earlier. But Schwarzenegger didn't need the box office totals in *Variety* to tell him that he needed to find something else to do with his life.

Schwarzenegger had taken a tentative step in that direction while filming *End of Days* in Los Angeles the year before. He summoned a Californian political consultant named Robert White to his trailer on the set outside St. Vincent de Paul Roman Catholic Church. As *Los Angeles Times* writer Joe Mathews would recount in his political biography, *The People's Machine*, Schwarzenegger observed that politics and movies were remarkably alike: both required a message that could capture an audience's imagination.

White suggested that Schwarzenegger use his popularity to make a run for governor of California. But the actor was reluctant. It wasn't that Schwarzenegger hadn't thought about entering politics. He had used his 1990 appointment to the President's Council on Physical Fitness and Sports as a political launching pad, meeting with the governors of all 50 states in an effort to create a national exercise program for children. He had also created the Inner-City Games in Los Angeles to help underprivileged children. Beyond that, Schwarzenegger subscribed to political journals to keep up on the ballot initiatives coming out of Sacramento. Still, there was still a part of him that held back, not quite sure if the time was right to make the leap.

An intimate of Schwarzenegger, a successful Ohio insurance executive named Jim Lorimer, was certain he would run eventually. Lorimer had been helping Schwarzenegger put on The Arnold Classic bodybuilding show for 26 years and was one of the few people who was able to appreciate how Schwarzenegger fused the worlds of politics, Hollywood, and bodybuilding. "Politics was something we talked about," he told Mathews. "I felt that was eventually one of the directions that he was going to go."

Indeed, Schwarzenegger was keeping his eyes on the 40,000 voters who streamed into Columbus's Veterans Memorial coliseum. They were socially conservative suburbanites with the kind of super-size desire for self-improvement that he was uniquely qualified to feed. A lucky few had tickets for the sold-out shows— two women's contests on Friday night and the all-male Arnold Classic Invitational on Saturday. But most were content to spend their time in the cavernous exhibition hall, filling empty shopping bags with the free samples that roughly 400 supplement vendors were happy to give out.

One of the attendees was a gravelly voiced man with a receding hairline and thinly manicured mustache who was a relative newcomer to the scene. He had only recently developed an interest in bodybuilding. Consequently, he had never attended The Arnold while Dan Duchaine held court.

The two men, in fact, had never met. But in one key respect, the strangers were mirror images of each other. Like Dan Duchaine, Victor Conte was a frustrated showman looking for a stage.

Victor Conte, Jr., was born on July 10, 1950, in the 120-degree heat of Death Valley, where his father owned a gas station beside a café run by his aunt. In 1954, the family moved to Lake Tahoe, briefly living in a tent on a construction site where Victor Sr. worked until the family finally settled in Fresno. In high school, Victor showed an early talent for track. But his real love was music. With two of his cousins, he formed a band and performed behind strippers at a notorious local bar called Arax's. One night, a bunch of goons walked in and gunned down the owner. After that, young Victor decided that his father might not have been wrong by suggesting that he go to the local community college. Conte studied accounting, but never gave up his bass, and eventually he found his way into a group that had just come off the road with the bluesman John Mayall.

The band released just one album in 1972, and over the next five years, Conte hung around the edges of the music industry getting work where he could. So he was thrilled when another opportunity for stardom presented itself. This one came courtesy of his older cousin Bruce, who had landed in the successful 10-piece funk group Tower of Power. Because of previous problems with two brothers who had been with the band, it had a rule against employing family members. But that was put aside when they heard Victor jam to an up-tempo number called "Can't You See" from the album *Oakland*. He started traveling the world as the band's bass player, making $3,000 a night.

Despite the pervasive drug culture of the San Francisco Bay Area in the 1970s, Conte would quip that he was one of the few not on drugs—"I was trying to work out with weights and do stuff." Seeing a void, he began assuming a role in the group's management. But his assertiveness reminded the others why they had passed the no-family rule in the first place. Early in 1979, the Conte cousins were told that it was time for them to leave.

Down the coast in Los Angeles, Dan Duchaine was creating a stir with the *Underground Steroid Handbook*. But in 1981, Conte was a 31-year-old married father of two daughters. He wasn't part of that scene. Instead, he had become interested in a trend that had become fashionable around the Bay Area: holistic medicine. With savings from his music career, he leased an office suite in the suburb of Millbrae and rented space to doctors while he sold vitamins from a storefront. (He figured that if the project failed, he could turn the space into a recording studio.)

Late in 1983, Conte found an opportunity that ended his music career for good. It involved an industrial machine that, among other things, was being used at Hughes Aircraft to analyze contaminants in oil drained from jets. An acquaintance held exclusive rights to the machine and suggested that with a little tinkering, it could be adapted for medical purposes. Conte already had a working knowledge of minerals. He decided that he could make a decent profit by using the machine to analyze blood for mineral deficiencies and then selling customers supplements to correct them.

Conte renamed the Millbrae Holistic Health Center the Bay Area Laboratory Cooperative and threw himself into selling the $40 tests. He convinced an Olympic judo coach and shot-putter to use them for mineral maintenance and sponsored two dozen athletes at the Seoul Games under the name BALCO Olympians. That kind of promotion didn't come cheap, personally or financially. Six figures worth of debt and a dozen IRS liens put pressure on his increasingly troubled marriage. After their separation, Conte even got a restraining order against his wife after a series of violent events, including an episode in which she tried to run him down with her car.[1]

In 1995, Conte turned to a Medicare billing scam that his older cousin, Michael, helped arrange. As explained by Lance Williams and Mark Fainaru-Wada in *Game of Shadows*, the cousins partnered with a Florida lab to charge geriatric patients for blood tests that they or their doctors never ordered. Federal attorneys ended up suing BALCO later for $1.8 million. (The case was settled in 2004 and the terms were undisclosed. Michael Conte pleaded guilty in 2000 to health care fraud, served 14 months, and was ordered to pay restitution.) One employee told the authors, "We immediately went from feast to absolutely nothing."

Still, Conte was too ambitious to be kept down for long. In the summer of 1995, his relentless networking skills brought him in contact with a speed coach who was working with the NFL's Bill Romanowski. The edgy linebacker embraced Conte's mineral tests and a friendship began. According to police records cited in *Game of Shadows*, Conte cemented it by selling Romanowski, who by then had signed with the Denver Broncos, human growth hormone. After a 117-tackle season, Romanowski arranged for Conte to visit the Broncos training camp in the spring of 1998. Wearing a white lab coat, Conte offered a blood test and free mineral workup to any player who wanted them.

San Francisco in the late 1990s was flush with money from the tech bubble. But the supplement industry was in the midst of its own boom. Seeing how much could be made, Conte came up with a pill that combined zinc and magnesium, along with a smooth sales pitch about how it helped high-performance athletes. Conte needed more than hype, though. He needed some kind of science on which he could hang his hat. Once again, Romanowski offered his assistance. He introduced his friend to the master marketer Bill Phillips.

---

1 Audrey Conte acknowledged in court that her behavior following the separation "left much to be desired."

The timing was intriguing. There wasn't anyone who understood the supplement business better than Phillips. But he was getting out. He had just released a movie, *Body of Work*, that showed him using a private jet to travel around the country, rewarding winners of his magazine's before-and-after fitness contest. (Even high-quality production values couldn't keep the vanity project from crumbling under the weight of Phillips's ego.) He was awaiting the publication of his book, *Body-for-LIFE*, and was negotiating to sell EAS. But Phillips still knew a good idea when he heard one. After Conte made a long and elaborate presentation, Phillips rewarded the Californian with $10,000 in seed money.

If anyone had a reason to be suspicious of Conte, it was Patrick Arnold. In the three years since he had arrived in Illinois to make his mark on the supplement world, he had succeeded in moving out of Dan Duchaine's shadow. He had his own business (with Stan Antosh and another partner) and was known on *misc.fitness.weights* as the new Guru. Not that he was living large. The money he expected to receive from Andro never quite materialized (all sides have different versions of why) and he was now residing in an old Victorian with moldy furniture, an oven that didn't work, and pipes that made the water feel hard and slick. Nonetheless, Arnold had what he wanted most: name recognition and a shot at making real money.

His new product, "Super Andro," was a gel-like version of the original that used a sugar-type molecule to solve a nagging problem: when it was swallowed, the steroid crystals that were released migrated to the liver, where enzymes attacked them like invading antibodies, turning the majority of crystals to waste. Arnold's advance made the crystals water soluble, allowing them to be absorbed more completely in the blood. Judging by the traffic at his company's booth at The Arnold, he had another hit on his hands. But Super Andro wasn't the most ingenious product he had come up with that year. His real breakthrough was a clear liquid that he simply called "The Stuff."

Victor Conte learned about The Stuff incidentally. The ex-musician had been using *misc.fitness.weights* as a personal bulletin board to hawk his zinc supplement, drawing the ire of regulars who saw him as a hack. One of the more voluble posters summed up the backlash by saying, "DIE, you piece of shit BALCO spammer." Arnold was more amused than threatened by the chatter, and after some early jousting, began a cordial exchange with Conte. When Conte asked him in a private e-mail about the clearance time of Andro, Arnold confided, "I have something that makes the whole issue of clearance times meaningless."

In the early 1960s, researchers at Wyeth Pharmaceuticals created a steroid that showed promise for treating dwarfism, but was too toxic to gain government approval. As a result, it sat relatively unnoticed in a textbook called *Androgens and Anabolic Agents: Chemistry and Pharmacology*. Arnold was leafing through the book one day in the mid-1990s when he stumbled across the compound. He immediately became fascinated by its design. In a 1995 post on *misc.fitness.weights*, he called it "one of the shining stars" of performance enhancers—an oral steroid that "[is] several of orders of magnitude ... more anabolic than methyl testosterone (the gold standard) and with only a small fraction of MT's androgenic potency."

Over the winter, after Arnold cooked up a small batch in his lab, he sent a vial to Conte in a plain brown box. In a few years, there would be talk about international conspiracies, dark intrigues, and tainted baseball statistics, but the reality was that it all came down to a guy without a working oven in his house and an ex-musician who spent his nights hustling himself on a nerdy online bulletin board.

Arnold's instructions were to take the mixture five times a week by dropping it beneath the tongue with a syringe. But Conte was wary about what he put into his body and started off slowly, taking the potion just twice a week at half of Arnold's recommended dosage.

Even at those lower levels, he could feel its effects. He bounced back from workouts quicker and didn't see any elevation in liver enzymes on his blood tests. Even better, there were no negative side effects like 'roid rages. It was exactly what Arnold had promised on the message board: "a shining star."

The first dose that Conte gave away went to his star client, Bill Romanowski. Another batch found its way to a legendary Ukrainian track coach who was working with Romanowski, Remi Korchemny. In short order, Korchemny offered it to several of his clients. By the time Patrick Arnold met Conte at The Arnold, the compound he had created as a hobby had started to take on a life of its own, and would play an even larger role at the Olympics in seven months.

SYDNEY, AUSTRALIA
September 26, 2000

The Opening Ceremony at the Olympics is always an event, and the Friday night pageant in Sydney was no exception. Don Catlin watched as Cathy Freeman, a gold medal hopeful and descendant of Aborigines, ascended the steps of the Olympic Stadium while they turned into a cascading waterfall. Then, Freeman literally walked on water en route to lighting a ring of fire that climbed brilliantly into the lit Olympic torch.

Before they had even begun, the Australian Freeman was already the darling of these Games. Close behind, though, was American track star Marion Jones, who was competing for something that no woman had ever attempted before: five gold medals in a single Games. In addition to her talent, Jones's cool beauty spoke to many constituencies—inner-city girls, black professionals, career women, track fans— that she had inked endorsement deals with nearly every sponsor that mattered: NBC, Nike, Gatorade, Panasonic, General Motors, AT&T, and Kellogg.

Gloating to *The New York Times*, United States Track & Field chief Craig Masback boasted that Jones had "already received more attention in terms of national television advertising campaigns than any athlete in history, more than Michael Jordan at one time."

But Jones also had a secret that involved her husband, shot-putter C.J. Hunter. In Sydney, the duo had the potential to be the first married couple in decades to vie for matching gold medals. But during the summer, Hunter failed four drug tests. The legal limit for nandrolone allowed by the International Association of Athletic Federations was two nanograms per milliliter. One of Hunter's urine samples contained 1,000 times that.

In a flurry of secret meetings with American track officials, Hunter was quietly presented with a deal: save the United States from embarrassment by withdrawing from the Games and his tests would not be made public. Four days before the opening ceremonies, Hunter did just that, citing an operation he had had on his left knee.

Once the Games began, Jones drew first blood in the 100-meter final. On a chilly, drizzly Saturday night at the Olympic Stadium, she sprang from the blocks with such astounding force that she won by the largest margin (.37 of a second) in the electronically timed era. The usual reserve with which she carried herself melted away as she hugged her mother and waived the flag of her Belize ancestry. To reporters, she said: "This is 16 years of believing and dreaming about this."

Within 36 hours, however, that dream turned fitful. Someone with knowledge of Hunter's failed tests leaked them to Sydney's *Daily Telegraph* and on Monday morning, the Olympic Village awoke to the story. No one was quicker to pounce than Dick Pound, the former aide to Juan Antonio Samaranch now on his maiden patrol as head of the new World Anti-Doping Agency. Pound, who once defended Ben Johnson, became the first public official to confirm the leaked report. "The United States should lead the way rather than being led, kicking and screaming, into being part of the solution," he acidly told reporters.

Masback, the head of USATF, could hardly have done more to play into Pound's hands. He held his own press conference to issue an official "no comment," making him seem just as obstructionist as Pound suggested.

With a crisis approaching, Jones's camp went into lockdown. Famed attorney Johnnie Cochran, who had once represented Jones for missing a drug test in high school (she appealed the proposed ban and won), was quickly summoned to help again. But that was only half the battle. They needed someone who looked good in a white lab coat, someone who could convince the public this report was all some horrible mistake.

Victor Conte was just getting up at 7 a.m. when C.J. Hunter arrived at his hotel room with an entourage. Since the spring, Conte's relationship with track coach Remi Korchemny was paying huge dividends. He had several new track clients and was picking up even more. During a meet in Europe, one of the newcomers, a relay gold medalist named Chryste Gaines, said on the phone to Conte: "There's someone here who wants to talk to you. His name is Tim Montgomery."

Montgomery was once one of the world's most promising 100-meter athletes, but his career was stalled. A couple of weeks earlier, he had tried and failed to make the U.S. Olympic team, finishing a woeful sixth in the finals. Conte and Montgomery chatted amiably and then talked again the next day, although this time it was with Montgomery's coach Trevor Graham listening in.

A tough-talking 37-year-old from Jamaica, Graham had his own agenda. He could do little for Montgomery before the Olympics. But Marion Jones was another story. After he assured himself that Conte was for real, Graham made a separate call with Jones's husband, Hunter, joining in. Conte's head spun when the two men broached the idea of him working with Jones. It was a huge leap; Marion was in a different league than Chryste Gaines.

Hunter became a critical link on the drug chain that went from Patrick Arnold in Illinois to Conte in California to Graham in North Carolina. According to Conte, he started sending drug packages to Graham, only to change course and send them directly to Hunter when he feared that Graham might be diverting them to his other clients. On the eve of the Sydney Olympics, the packages included Norbolethone, synthetic EPO, insulin, and human growth hormone. (Hunter reportedly told investigators that he watched Jones take the liquid version by placing two drops on her tongue and helped her inject the EPO into her buttocks. Jones denied these allegations.)

But Hunter had a request of his own: he needed help explaining his four failed drug tests. With the help of Patrick Arnold, Conte zeroed in on an iron pill that Hunter had bought in Rome earlier that summer. It was made by a New York firm that also packaged 19-norandrostenedione for clients. Conte called the plant's manager and learned that it mixed both products in the same room. Considering how dusty it got, he told Hunter that it was at least possible that a steroid-filled mist had seeped into the vitamin vat and contaminated it.

The shot-putter chose to withdraw from the Games rather than mount that defense. But now that the whole thing had spilled into the public's eye, he barged into Conte's hotel room with his sponsors in tow. "Tell them what you found," he said.

Conte told the story amid much head nodding. Before he knew it, he was being whisked to another hotel to meet Johnnie Cochran. There, he told the story for a second time. The defense attorney looked at him carefully. "Okay," Cochran said. "You're the guy. We have a press conference full of people who are waiting to hear what C.J. has to say. You're going to explain all this to them."

At that, Conte was put into a waiting van and sped off to pick up Jones so they could address the world's media.

Don Catlin was just settling into a seat in the ballroom when Hunter arrived hand in hand with Jones. He had watched Jones win the gold the prior Saturday night. Now he was watching as she walked in with her husband amid a swirl of flash bulbs and took the microphone first.

"I am here pretty much to show my complete support for my husband," Jones began. "I have total and complete respect for him and believe the legal system will do what's needed to clear his name." Then she begged the press to respect her privacy and kissed Hunter before exiting.

On stage alone, Hunter apologized for the distractions he had caused to his wife. Dabbing one eye with a tissue and sniffling, he said, "The reason I throw is so I can travel around the world with my wife for free. Track and field has never been that important to me—not to the point that I would do something like this. I don't know what has happened and I don't know how it has happened, but how it may affect me is the least of my concerns."

No surprises there, Catlin thought. Hunter was going for the sympathy play. But then something truly surprising happened. A stout man with a gravely voice appeared out of nowhere to explain that Hunter's four failed tests were due to iron supplements he had bought in Rome. Catlin had a short list of people he expected to see in situations such as these, and this man—what was his name, Monte?—wasn't one of them. If Hunter had tested at 10 times above the legal limit, Catlin might be able to accept the defense. Even 20 times. But a 1,000 times? People had to see that. Then again, why should they? Sports fans kept track of box scores, not periodic tables.

Catlin left the ballroom wondering about the newcomer. He seemed to be smart, or at least smart enough to work his way into the biggest press conference of the Olympics. Perhaps it was time to add Victor Conte to his list of usual suspects.

BURLINGAME, CALIFORNIA
November 17, 2000

The morning edition of the *San Francisco Chronicle* carried the latest news about the Presidential election of November 7. Though the networks had called Florida for Vice President Al Gore early in the evening, Texas Governor George W. Bush had staged one of the most remarkable political comebacks in history by midnight to win the state by a mere 300 votes. Ten days later, a stunned Gore was still refusing to concede; Broward County election workers were recounting 588,000 ballots by hand while more than 2,500 more overseas ballots were being tabulated.

Tim Montgomery, meanwhile, was hoping to wage his own improbable comeback as he waited in his San Francisco hotel for Victor Conte to pick him up. Having failed to earn a spot on the 2000 Olympic team, Montgomery flew into town to take Conte up on an offer: Conte would give him exclusive access to drugs that would make Montgomery the world's fastest man if Montgomery endorsed his ZMA supplement.

One of the people whom Conte had invited to join them was Charlie Francis. Since his career had disintegrated with Ben Johnson in Seoul, Francis was playing the role of martyred wise man. In the nine years since he had testified before the Dubin Commission, Francis had stuck around Toronto, hiding in plain sight and regularly attending track meets. While he told curiosity seekers that he was making his living training wealthy businessmen, the reality was that coaching advice was still widely sought. It galled Francis that he had to give it in the shadows; if he were ever caught he would be publicly disowned. But that's how the game went. Hiring Charlie Francis was just one more thing that a track star had to do in secret.

Another of Conte's recruits was a Yugoslavian bodybuilder, Milos Sarcev. Having won the 1989 Mr. Universe title, Sarcev had been hanging around the Bay Area for a decade and was a charter member of Pat Arnold's chemical circle. In February, Sarcev was shopping for drugs and asked if oral trenbolone was the "miracle drug" that Arnold had been boasting about.

"No, the miracle stuff is called Norbolethone," Arnold answered. "I could get about four grams of this stuff to you right away: $100 per gram. The oral tren stuff is still an unknown because no one else has really tried it in a controlled manner [someone clean taking it by itself]. That stuff is 200 bucks a gram and I do have a gram made up."

When Graham arrived a day after Montgomery, the table was set to build the perfect athletic beast. Everybody had some legitimate role to play: Francis came with a technical critique about how Montgomery, a blistering midrace runner, needed to find more power out of the blocks. Sarcev took him into a gym in the back room for an upper-body workout to improve his shoulder strength. And Conte had designed a mineral program.

But the most important player wasn't there. Patrick Arnold was more than 2,000 miles away in Illinois, replacing the Norbolethone that Montgomery was getting with an improved drug that would take them, and the sports world itself into uncharted new waters— the kind that his mentor, Dan Duchaine, would have loved.

14

A BULLY PULPIT

May 1, 2001 - November 11, 2001

COLORADO SPRINGS, COLORADO

May 1, 2001

Terrence Madden, debonair and silver-haired, couldn't wait for this first anniversary to be over. Precisely one year earlier, the ex-bond trader had walked into an empty office in Colorado Springs, hung his Notre Dame law degree on the wall, and began work as the head of the United States Anti-Doping Agency. A thick binder that sat on his desk gave the outlines of what was expected of him. It was a task force report commissioned by the U.S. Olympic Committee that dealt with a radical idea: What would happen if drug penalties were no longer the responsibility of individual sports, but were put in the hands of an independent agency? The idea had certain legal advantages: chief executives in sports such as swimming or track & field would no longer be tempted to favor their stars; punishment would be money-blind. As the report concluded, "The creation of an organization that is independent from the USOC will enhance international credibility of US anti-doping efforts."

Madden was intimately familiar with the conclusions because he had worked on them. After getting his law degree, he had spent a year in the Dallas DA's office, only to discover that he hated the grind of revolving-door justice. He traded the courtroom for the stock car pace of the Chicago Board of Trade and by his mid-40s had made enough to enjoy an early retirement and a move to Colorado. Madden briefly dabbled in mergers and acquisitions, sizing up banks that were ripe for takeovers. But that gave way to an ever more eclectic job when he was invited to run the national governing body for USA Badminton. As a sports fanatic, he agreed and was barely a year into the job when the president of the U.S. Olympic Committee, Bill Hybl, recruited him to become his chief of staff. Under Hybl, Madden served as a liaison to the task force that ultimately created USADA.

In November 1999, Madden flew to Chicago to address nine men and women who had volunteered to serve as the agency's initial board of directors. As was typical in such situations, Madden was direct and to the point. From now on, they would be responsible for drug testing athletes in all Olympic sports. The USOC had set an ambitious goal for their first year: they would have to process 5,000 tests in 45 sports. And it went without saying that their work had to be above reproach. "There are a lot of things you're going to be doing for the first time," he cautioned. First on the list was choosing someone who could keep it all running.

As he thought about the workload, he told himself, "I pity the guy they pick. So many things can go wrong; this thing has failure written all over it."

They picked Madden.

The 50-year-old tried to go about his work quietly, discreetly making calls and building a staff. But political rivalries have a way of interfering with major structural change and this was no different. When the USOC's chief drug tester learned that he was being shunted aside, he refused to go quietly. After trying and failing to negotiate a seven-figure severance package for himself, the doctor, Wade Exum, filed a multimillion-dollar discrimination suit. (It was dismissed and a new suit was eventually settled for an undisclosed amount.) He added to the drama by making explosive accusations that his superiors routinely meddled in his affairs to protect their star athletes.

Olympic veterans had already suspected that the big names got preferential treatment; Exum's charges just affirmed their deep-seated cynicism. Madden felt it when he flew to Sydney on a fact-finding mission before the 2000 Olympic Games. The Australians were some of the best drug testers in the world. "I could tell by the way they looked at me that they were wondering if this was going to be the same old story with the USA," Madden would recall.

Some good ideas came out of the trip. The Aussies asked their athletes to give advance notice of their whereabouts so they could always be tracked. Using that as a starting point, Madden went one better with a three-strike rule: any American who wasn't where he or she promised to be on three different occasions within an 18-month rolling period would be treated the same as if he or she had tested positive.

Still, the past continued to cloud the future. No sooner had Madden returned to Colorado than the news about C.J. Hunter's positive drug tests exploded into the news. White House drug czar Barry McCaffrey was quick to use the affair to question whether Madden's close ties with the USOC would allow him to be a truly independent figure.

At dinner with his wife and three kids, he warned that things were about to get rough. "Daddy's going to try to do a good job," Madden said, "but some people are probably going to say some pretty bad things about me."

During their first six months, Madden's staff paid surprise visits to 319 athletes in sports ranging from biathlon, bobsledding, cycling, judo, rowing, shooting, speed skating, swimming, tae kwon do, track, triathlon, water polo, weightlifting, and wrestling. Another 1,181 tests were done during competitions. It was a dizzying baptism into the world of elite sport.

But following that—after all the tough talk, all the headlines—the first USADA catch wasn't a gold medalist or a millionaire. It was an overachieving 16-year-old fencer who was also studying cello, cooking, and Latin. With all she had going on, she had fallen behind on her schoolwork and had taken her sister's attention deficit disorder medication so she could pull an all-nighter. At the U.S. Fencing Junior Olympics in February, she tripped the drug test for an elevated level of amphetamine.

The cardinal rule that governs USADA's work is known as *strict liability*: If it's in your body, you're guilty. But how could this case not warrant extenuating circumstances? How could this be what USADA was supposed to be doing with its $9 million opening budget?

The girl's father called and begged Madden to be reasonable. After much pleading, Madden said the best he could do was reduce the two-year suspension to one. On his first anniversary, he approved a press release that announced the 16-year-old cellist as his first catch.

CARMEL, INDIANA
May 2001

Bruce Kneller received hundreds of e-mails a day from a broad cross-section of Steroid Nation—high school kids, desk jockeys, college athletes, gym rats. They all wanted help decoding the thicket of chemical names and claims that came spilling out over the Internet. For the most part, they reflected the retail end of the nation, which is where Kneller had set up shop. But every so often, he got an e-mail about someone working on the other side of the business—the private label end where designer steroids were made for a select few.

And it was one of those e-mails that had caught his eye. The sender was asking him about a brand-new drug making the underground rounds called tetrahydrogestrinone. Kneller went to his copy of *Androgens and Anabolic Agents: Chemistry and Pharmacology* and found a two-dimensional diagram that matched it exactly. There were at most a handful of people who had the knowledge and ability to synthesize THG, and he was one of them.

Another? "This has to be Pat Arnold," he thought. "What is he up to?"

ATLANTA

May 20, 2001

Barry Bonds didn't notice the 33,696 fans rising to their feet, or so he would say. He was generally indifferent to what those around him thought, so maybe it was true. Or maybe the man who kept the world at bay was just waiting for the right moment to let it in. If so, this was that moment.

After starting April with the second worst slump of his career, Bonds had found more than a groove. He had found a way to bend time itself. The patience he displayed at the plate might have seemed serene if it weren't so naked and predatory. His pitch selections were more than smart. They were brushstrokes, each adding another layer to an emerging masterpiece. Coming into the day's game, he had 20 home runs in 32 games. Three of them came the evening before in a rain-delayed stunner in Atlanta.

A first inning shot off John Burkett this afternoon made it five homers in the last three games. Then, after the Braves walked him twice, he launched an even more impressive 436-footer over the centerfield wall. Bonds was rewarded with the rarest sign of respect for a hitter: an out-of-town standing-O as he crossed home plate. Braves manager Bobby Cox added his own exclamation point when he observed that Bonds was "playing, honest to God, like he's 27."

The main reason for Bonds's career renaissance had to do with his trainer, Greg Anderson, a former college player who operated out of a gym just two blocks from Victor Conte's BALCO. After Conte's efforts in Sydney, Anderson was more than a little intrigued about what his neighbor could do for his client. In the fall of 2000—at the very moment that Conte was plotting how to turn Tim Montgomery into a world champion—Anderson wrangled an introduction.

Conte had barely shaken off the jet lag from Sydney—indeed, had barely gotten over having Montgomery and Marion Jones as clients—when the doors to Major League Baseball swung wide open.

In later years, it would be fashionable to say that baseball didn't have a rule against taking steroids, so no one who used them could truly be blamed. That reasoning is incorrect and facile on several levels. First, taking steroids without a doctor's prescription was illegal. And second, baseball did have a rule. A memo issued by then-commissioner Fay Vincent in 1991 and unearthed by *ESPN The Magazine*'s Tom Farrey explicitly included steroids on the banned list. It was reissued six years later by Vincent's successor, Bud Selig. What is more accurate to say is that Selig failed to enforce his own rules. As a result, Anderson was free to give his star client access to a BALCO club that was getting perilously crowded.

MOSCOW

July 13, 2001

Tu Mingde was in a surprisingly good mood, considering that the question being put to him was whether a nation that recently had executed 1,791 of its own citizens deserved to host an Olympics. The co-secretary general of China's effort to land the 2008 Summer Games smiled before the international press, to show how warmly they would be greeted in his country if it won the bidding. "Thank you for your question," he said gamely.

Tu had every reason to feel confident. One hundred and nineteen members of the International Olympic Committee were going to be voting tomorrow morning on a host city for 2008, and China was a lock. Eight years earlier, its leaders were humiliated when Sydney pulled a surprise upset in its quest to host the 2000 Games. But the world's most populous nation was on the brink of getting a multibillion-dollar make-up call.

Of course, there was ample reason to oppose the move, which the U.S. Congress did by introducing a symbolic resolution. The main one was China's human rights record. According to a report issued by Amnesty International, the communist leadership was using its sports stadiums for bizarre public humiliation spectacles in which criminals were jeered at by average citizens before being put to death.

On a more prosaic level, there was the question of China's doping program, which Don Catlin was deeply familiar with. In the early 1990s, he had been asked to take part in a fact-finding trip to Beijing. As soon as Catlin arrived, Chinese officials tried to take him to a training center in the far western part of the country, hours away by plane. Catlin saw through the offer as a ruse to get him out of the capital. So he politely declined and asked if he could see the main analysis lab in Beijing.

His hosts complied, but Catlin immediately got the feeling that the lab where they had led him wasn't the one he wanted to see. He knew how busy his lab was on an average day. This one should have been twice as busy with all that was going on in Chinese athletics. Yet it had a stilted, almost picturesque air. Some beakers literally had coats of dust on them. Though Catlin couldn't prove it, he had a nagging sense that the real lab was being kept from his investigative eyes.

Over the next few years, China's reputation for state-sponsored doping grew worse. A group of female long-distance runners nicknamed Ma's Army (because they were coached by the legendary Ma Junren) raised eyebrows by setting world records in the 1,500 meters, 3,000 meters, and 10,000 meters over one week in the fall of 1993. Because China had little history in the sport, Ma tried to deflect scrutiny by giving credit to a supplement regimen that included turtle blood and caterpillar fungus. Crediting exotic supplements for his success became harder to do the next year, when China took 12 of 16 medals at the world swimming championships, as well as at the Asian Games a few months later, when 11 of its athletes flunked drug tests.

By the 2000 Olympics in Sydney, Chinese Olympic officials understood that they couldn't keep ducking the obvious, not if China wanted to host the Olympics Games. In an unprecedented move, Ma was removed from China's Olympic team, along with six of his runners. In all, 27 Chinese athletes were told they would not travel to Sydney. "Some of them are dropped due to suspicious blood test results," He Huixian, a spokesman, announced in a moment of unprecedented candor.

But there was one doping problem that he wasn't addressing: the one caused by his country's fast-growing pharmaceutical industry. Without antisteroid laws like the ones in America to hold them back China's factories were producing high-quality steroids that easily found their way into the international underground. From his lab in Champaign, Illinois, for instance, Patrick Arnold was regularly wiring $650 to Chinese bank accounts to pay for the raw materials he needed to experiment with THG.

That was a subject the Chinese weren't eager to embrace. Fortunately, they didn't have to do so. On July 14, the IOC announced that Beijing had won the 2008 Games.

ST. LOUIS

November 11, 2001

Mark McGwire would have given anything to have had that one last at bat. It was bad enough that he had to watch Barry Bonds shatter the single-season home run record that he had set just three years earlier. Since then, McGwire seemed to be living in dog years. His right knee had required surgery. His back ached. Most of all, his spirit seemed weary. Bonds, meanwhile, was living in some bizarre parallel universe. At the age of 37, he had gotten stronger as the season went along and won a record-breaking fourth MVP award.

What was McGwire thinking? Did he see Bonds as a fellow traveler? If so, he must have suspected that Bonds would eventually crash the way he was crashing now. McGwire wasn't able to get down low enough to drive the ball the way he once did and the result was a .187 average with 118 strikeouts in 299 at bats. During a thrilling season in which his Cardinals battled the Houston Astros for first place, McGwire sulked around the clubhouse, making his teammates uncomfortable.

No one defended McGwire more than St. Louis manager Tony La Russa. But in the end, there was nowhere La Russa could hide his veteran during the fifth game of the National League Division Series in Arizona. With the game tied 1-1 in the ninth, Jim Edmonds led with a single up the middle, bringing up McGwire. Not long ago, La Russa would have expected magic. But McGwire had struck out three times that night. La Russa sized up his slugger and decided to pull him for a rookie, Kerry Robinson. The message had been delivered. Big Mac was no longer The Man.

Now, a depressed McGwire was sending his own message. Late on this Sunday night, a fax machine at the Bristol, Connecticut, offices of ESPN spit out the following statement:

"After a considerable discussion with those close to me, I have decided not to sign the [contract] extension, as I am unable to perform at a level equal to the salary the organization would be paying me. I believe I owe it to the Cardinals and the fans of St. Louis to step aside, so a talented free agent can be brought in as the final piece of what I expect can be a world championship-caliber team. So I am walking away from the game that has provided me opportunities, experiences, memories and friendships to fill 10 lifetimes. For years I have said my motivation for playing wasn't for fame and fortune, but rather the love of competing. Baseball is a team sport and I have been lucky enough to contribute to the success of some great teams. I want to thank the St. Louis Cardinal organization."

The people "close to" McGwire apparently didn't include anyone from the Cardinals. Despite his warm words, he failed to give the front office advance notice about his intentions. The snub would lead to considerable armchair analyzing. Was McGwire trying to send a signal to La Russa after the benching? Was he too depressed to think clearly? Or did he just want to disappear as quickly as possible, and take the secrets of an era with him?

15

THE SCIENTIST STRIKES BACK

February 23, 2002 - September 15, 2002

SALT LAKE CITY

February 23, 2002

Don Catlin was tired of playing defense. With the 2002 Winter Games on his home turf, he was once again being called upon to run the whole Olympic drug-testing operation, just as he had done in Los Angeles in 1984 and Atlanta in 1996. This time around, however, he had come up with a surprise.

For years, Catlin had been tracking a drug called darbepoetin. It was an exciting breakthrough on the cancer front because, like EPO, it could help patients bounce back from chemotherapy by spurring the production of red blood cells, yet its effects lasted longer. Unfortunately, darbepoetin was also making the rounds of the sports underground. In Spain, where it was marketed under the brand name NESP, athletes were paying patients with prescriptions for access to the drug. Normally, that would have irritated the hell out of Catlin—another sign of how hard it was for him to stay a step ahead of the cheaters—but he had an idea.

Two years earlier in Sydney, his French colleagues had debuted a test for EPO and failed spectacularly. Out of 300 samples, not a single person was caught. That left a lot of scientists having to mutter an embarrassed explanation: Since EPO breaks down very quickly in urine (usually within three days), it takes luck to catch a user—even with a good test.

The French scientists vowed to improve the test for Salt Lake, and in the summer of 2001, Catlin sent a team to Paris to learn from their work. The test was immensely complicated, but Catlin believed it could be adapted for NESP.

He needed two things first: a reference version of the drug and a sample from someone who had taken it. The former was resolved itself with a call to Amgen, the California drug company that made it. The second part was trickier. Catlin couldn't very well advertise in *Cheater's Quarterly.* Luckily, a clinical trial for cancer patients was underway at the UCLA Medical Center. And while it took seven months for the sample to arrive, it finally did on February 7—the day before the Olympics began. Catlin's dry run on the reference sample was an unqualified success. When the French method was applied to the synthetic darbepoetin, it showed up clearly on the sample.

Shortly before the opening ceremonies, Catlin approached the IOC's new president, a progressive Belgian doctor named Jacques Rogge. Placing his finger on the three clear bands in his test sample, he said, "It's darbepoetin. I'm convinced this test will work."

"Can you win at CAS?" Rogge asked, referring to the Court for Arbitration in Sport, a kind of Supreme Court for doping cases, where any athlete who challenged his findings would surely bring an appeal. Catlin said he would stake his reputation on it.

"Okay," Rogge replied.

By Thursday, February 21, Catlin was starting to feel less certain about his prediction. He had conducted hundreds of tests, but had not turned up a positive.

Meanwhile, an hour's drive from Salt Lake, in a tiny village called Soldiers Hollow, a cross-country skier named Johann Muehlegg was celebrating. Muehlegg had spent most of his life in Germany, racking up a modest record in his sport. But now, after deciding to join the Olympic team of his native Spain, he seemed reborn. Spain isn't exactly a traditional power in skiing; it had won only two winter medals before Salt Lake. Muehlegg, however, was on fire. He had won two medals and was a favorite in the 50-kilometer endurance race that was to be run on Saturday. Things were going so well for him, in fact, that he didn't seem the least concerned when an Olympic drug tester knocked on his door at 10 p.m. and asked him to come to a doping control station to give a sample.

The next afternoon, Catlin was in his Salt Lake command center when a technician came running over to him. "Dr. Catlin," he said. "I think you should see this."

Once Catlin laid eyes on the computer screen, he knew what he had: the thick bands on the top of the sample were unmistakable. It was darbepoetin. At that exact moment, someone snapped a photo of Catlin. He had a tight smile and was holding two thumbs up.

Science moves slowly, but time was the last thing that Catlin had, especially because two more positives came in later that night. In a dizzying 36 hours, he checked his findings, consulted with Olympic lawyers, and put together a formal report for the IOC. Then he held his breath. It wasn't so long ago that the IOC's old medical czar, Prince Alexandre de Mérode of Belgium, looked him in the eye and declined to act on the five positives that Catlin had found in Atlanta.

But Juan Samaranch and his crowd were gone from the IOC, replaced by Rogge. On the eve of the closing ceremonies, Rogge received Catlin's report and took a deep breath himself. He was being asked to strip three athletes—Muehlegg and two Russian skiers—of their medals, based almost solely on Catlin's reputation for scrupulousness. The easiest thing would have been for Rogge to say the whole affair needed further study. Instead, he went in the opposite direction. He announced Catlin's findings and stripped the three athletes.

The reaction was volcanic. The head of Russia's Olympic Committee questioned the legality of even introducing a surprise test like the one Catlin had used. "The Olympics should not be a field for experiments," he said.

But Rogge's decision held. Don Catlin had just scored one for the offense.

CHULA VISTA, CALIFORNIA

March 14, 2002

The U.S. Olympic Training Center's 155-acre complex spreads over rolling hills that are manicured to nurture the hopes of the 4,000 athletes who reside there. One of them, a 34-year-old cyclist named Tammy Thomas, had been as close as anybody to representing America in the 2000 Olympics in track cycling, a sport in which riders travel on a banked indoor track at 40 mph without brakes.

Her only real rival was a veteran Utah racer named Chris Witty. In certain circles, they were coarsely referred to as beauty and the beast; while Witty had schoolgirl looks, Thomas had the unflattering profile of a woman who had tested positive for excessive testosterone. At their showdown at the national time trials, Thomas beat Witty by a .025-second margin. Unfortunately, because of her failed tests, USA Cycling refused to award her the Sydney spot and declared Witty the overall favorite.

Thomas may have been raised among Southern belles in the Mississippi Delta, but she didn't go quietly. She filed a lawsuit (the first of many) that led a judge to order a rideoff between the women. When Witty boycotted the event, Thomas raced alone. But her solo victory was short lived. The win was overturned when it was revealed that she had flunked her drug test at the earlier trials. With her case falling apart, Thomas surrendered her legal challenge in exchange for getting a customary four-year suspension reduced to one year.

Among the friends she leaned on for support in this period was a female bodybuilder named Kelsey Dalton. The two biked regularly together and Thomas even sold her one of her used machines. The friendship might have gone unnoticed except for one detail: Kelsey Dalton was the girlfriend of Patrick Arnold.

As the sun was starting to set on this spring afternoon in Chula Vista, Thomas had just returned from a grueling daylong workout in the hills. Since serving her one-year suspension, she had won a silver medal at the 2001 world championships in Belgium and felt strong about the coming season.

A urine collector for the U.S. Anti-Doping Agency knocked on her door. Thomas had been through the ritual enough that she let the collector into her dormitory and did what was expected, without much fuss. She was certain that this time around, she had nothing to worry about.

LOS ANGELES
March 18, 2002

Sometimes it's what you *don't* see in a urine sample that leads you to be suspicious.

Since his triumph in Salt Lake, Don Catlin had become a minor media celebrity. Reporters who had never paid attention to his work were now calling for interviews. But on this afternoon, he was back to the daily grind, leafing through the hundreds of graphs generated by his gas-chromatography/mass-spectrometry machines. And one result drew his attention.

The reading for testosterone in a female athlete was way too low. It was almost as if she wasn't producing any of the hormone. Maybe this person had an unusually low natural output. Or maybe Athlete X (Catlin didn't know her name) was taking so much synthetic testosterone that it had shut down her natural supply.

After ordering a second, more thorough test, Catlin turned up a signature that resembled a steroid called norethandrolone. Now he was really intrigued. Norethandrolone wasn't a molecule you saw every day. Eager to know more, he entered a molecular diagram of it into a medical database and retrieved a list of all related chemicals. Sitting at the top of the list was another drug, Norbolethone.

He soon began surfing the underground chat rooms and message boards to see who else was talking about it. For such a supposedly secret drug, no one seemed to be particularly cautious. Charlie Francis wrote glowingly about it on a Web site in 2001, using the trade name Genabol. And Patrick Arnold's own posts on *misc.fitness.weights* linked him in the plainest way.

Just as he had done with darbepoetin, Catlin called the drug company that originated it, Wyeth, and asked for a sample. As it turned out, Wyeth's head of research spent his summers at a family-oriented camp run by Catlin's brother in the Adirondacks and followed his work. He wrote back to say that he couldn't find a sample in Wyeth's archives because the drug was so old. Catlin's next step was to call one of the leaders of the Wyeth research team that had worked on Norbolethone. Now 69 years old and retired, the scientist couldn't have been more surprised to hear that Catlin had found evidence that it was back.

"You say you've found Norbolethone?" he repeated. "No, that's quite impossible. There's none of it left. I'm sure what you've found was caused by a birth control pill. They have similar fingerprints, you know." Catlin knew. The birth control drug Levonorgestrel contained some of the same molecular markers as Norbolethone. But they weren't a precise match.

"Thank you for your time," Catlin said.

A couple of months later, an employee at Wyeth phoned the UCLA lab to say that a small sample of the drug had been located in their archives. When it arrived, Catlin eagerly put it through his GC/MS machine. It was a perfect match with Athlete X.

But now that he had solved one mystery, Catlin was faced with another, larger one. Did Wyeth have a rogue chemist in its midst, digging around in the old vaults? Or was someone else rooting through Wyeth's past?

CALI, COLOMBIA

June 23, 2002

Now that Tammy Thomas had worked her way up to second in the world, all seemed to be forgiven with USA Cycling. She had been selected to represent the United States in the World Cup in Cali, Colombia, and she rewarded its faith by winning the 500-meter time trial and finishing second in the sprint. Her comeback was all but complete.

That was, if she could just hold on a little bit longer. On April 10, she had come to the end of another long practice day when she received her mail. Amid the usual fare, one envelope stuck out. It was a Federal Express pouch. Looking at the return address, her heart sank. It was from the U.S. Anti-Doping Agency.

Don Catlin reported his finding as a positive drug test, and the prosecutorial machinery operated by USADA was kicking in. The "Dear Ms. Thomas" letter inside informed her that:

> *"Your urine sample collected at Chula Vista, California, on March 14, 2002, was sent to the IOC accredited laboratory at the University of California at Los Angeles for analysis. The laboratory has reported that your sample contains the prohibited substance Norbolethone (Genabol), an anabolic androgenic steroid.*

*The laboratory's positive A-sample report and its docu-
mentation package are enclosed with this letter. At this
time, you have the right to accept the laboratory results
in order to avoid further delay in the adjudication of
your case.... If you choose not to accept the A-sample
results, your B-sample will be opened at the UCLA laboratory on April 24."*

Thomas chose the latter. The result was confirmed.

The prospect of a doping hearing threw Patrick Arnold into a
new panic. On May 1, he wrote to Victor Conte, saying, "I know
the girl they just snagged for Norbolethone. I saw her tests and
everything. She is trying to fight it and I am advising her technically
how to do it. Needless to say, if you know anyone taking the stuff
who is subject to testing, then tell them to stop." Thomas wasn't
even supposed to be using Norbolethone. More than a year ago, he
had advised her to replace it with a newer compound, THG.

In an official reply, Thomas said that the results were caused by
the birth control pills she was taking. But Terry Madden at USADA
wasn't persuaded. If he could go after a 16-year-old fencer who had
taken an ADD medication, he wasn't about to back off a known
doper—much less one who was eligible for a lifetime ban. For the
moment, he was bound by secrecy rules. He couldn't announce
anything until his review board approved the charges he wanted to
file. So Thomas waved to the Cali crowd, hoping that her personal
chemist would get her out of this one, too.

COLORADO SPRINGS, COLORADO
August 20, 2002

Until the Tammy Thomas hearing, Don Catlin had begun to
question whether USADA was really worth all the time and money
that was being poured into it. He had been called to testify in at

least a dozen hearings since the agency opened its doors. And for the most part, the athletes he was testifying against seemed to be kids who had made stupid mistakes. He believed every word of one woman who insisted that the nandrolone in her system had come from a contaminated supplement. But what could he do? He had to testify as to what the tests showed. As he would recall later:

"All our energy and resources were going out to the small cases that didn't have any effect. I'd sit in hearings, watching kids' moms and dads sitting there crying. And there I am, the big bad guy, saying, 'Throw 'em out.' And I didn't like it. Not one bit. These weren't people who set out to break the rules. The longer I testified, the crappier I felt."

But as he walked into the hearing room to testify in front of Thomas, he put those thoughts aside. Norbolethone was a real cheater's drug. And he had caught the cyclist with it, hands down.

With Thomas burning a hole in him with her eyes, he began his testimony. Thomas and her attorneys had come with a litany of complaints: that an academic paper Catlin filed about his research into Norbolethone turned her drug test into a "human research project"; that the seals on her urine samples hadn't been checked as closely as the rules required; that it took an inappropriately long time, four days, for the sample that she had given to reach his lab.

He patiently replied to each charge in the confident tone of a man who had never lost a case in court, finally hanging her with a simple statement of fact: Norbolethone looked like Norbolethone, not like birth control. Any argument otherwise was, at best, a "theoretical possibility."

His testimony was enough to convince the three arbitrators hearing her case to vote for a lifetime ban. It was the first ban ever meted out by USADA, and Madden thanked him for all his hard work. But for Catlin, there remained the gnawing sense of a job not quite done. Her chemist was still out there.

PARIS
September 15, 2002

Patrick Arnold wished he could undo what he had started. Too many records were falling, and too many questions being asked. After failing to break the 10-second mark for two years, Tim Montgomery suddenly did it six times in 2001, including a gaudy 9.95 time in Eugene, Oregon, which won him his first-ever USA Outdoor title. (The women's champion that day was another BALCO client, Chryste Gaines.) Each time Montgomery broke a new barrier en route to becoming the second-ranked sprinter in the world, Conte excitedly called Patrick Arnold. "This is great!" he would say with almost childlike glee. "Can you believe it?"

No, Arnold couldn't. He hadn't told his business partners what he had done, much less his family or friends. As a result, the bigger that Conte got, the more vulnerable Arnold felt. He liked Conte; they had fun when they met at The Arnold or Mr. Olympia shows. But as he would say in an interview with this writer years later, "Victor gave it to too many people and the playing field was getting too uneven. I got into this business because I wanted to become the guy that people who bought supplements could trust. Instead, I was helping people I didn't care about. I just didn't want to go down that road anymore."

While Conte and Montgomery had parted ways over an allegedly unpaid debt—Conte claimed that he had loaned Montgomery $25,000—Montgomery was still rising, thanks to the supply of THG that had lasted him well into the year. Montgomery had recently finished first in meets in Zurich, Brussels, Paris, and Stockholm. Arnold, meanwhile, already had trouble sleeping at night. But he found a whole new reason to stay awake with this morning's *Chicago Tribune*. The front page of the sports section reported: "A new fastest human at 9.78. Montgomery sets 100-meter mark." Reading the first two paragraphs of the story by reporter Philip Hersh made the chemist feel ill:

> *"Tim Montgomery has complained all summer about not getting the financial respect from meet promoters he thought was due the world's second-fastest sprinter. He refused to run races at Athens in June and Berlin eight days ago because the appearance fees were too low.*
>
> *Montgomery changed all that in 9.78 seconds Saturday at the Grand Prix Final in Paris. Not only did his world record for the 100 meters earn him an instant $250,000, it had the potential to triple his appearance fee to an estimated $60,000 per meet next season."*

"This was a lark that I did on the side, not my life," Arnold would say. "That was when I went from feeling, 'Hey, this is kinda neat' to 'This is wrong.' Victor was all excited. But it wasn't a game anymore to me. I wasn't taking any pride in it. I wanted out."

The trouble was, Arnold couldn't get out. The THG was so potent that Montgomery had all he needed. All the chemist could do was wait.

16

THE TWO ARNOLDS

February 18, 2003 - September 3, 2003

The NFL was the first professional sports league to routinely test for steroids, and as a result had built a reputation as a dedicated partner in the doping fight. But on any given Sunday, a good portion of the league was still probably hopped up on something. Unlike in baseball, where muscle enhancement was a matter of will and greed, in the NFL where super-sized men collided at supernatural speeds, it was a matter of survival.

All of which led to this barren stretch of industrial detritus near Douglas International Airport in Charlotte, where an unassuming, round-faced doctor named James Shortt was doing his part to help the Carolina Panthers become Super Bowl champions.

On a cool February morning, tight end Wesley Walls pulled up to Shortt's red-brick office in search of help. After five Pro Bowl seasons, Walls was nearly at the end of his career. His team's coach, John Fox, had spent the prior season retooling the offense, preaching run and not pass. In the new scheme, Walls had to do more blocking than catching. Since he was gifted with his hands, not his hits, he had become a drag on the team's salary cap. The Panthers were faced with the prospect of owing him $1 million in bonus money and his 2003 salary was going to cost the team four times as much. Even though Walls had offered to restructure his contract, the writing was on the wall: he was a dead man walking on two surgically repaired knees.

Shortt had billed himself as a "life extensionist," but his waiting room smelled an awful lot like death. Seated in a half-dozen leather recliners were patients with, among other ailments, Lyme disease, prostate cancer, and multiple sclerosis. Shortt had the MS patients hooked up to IV drips that pumped out a strong brew of hydrogen peroxide. The treatment was controversial at best, dangerous at worst. But Shortt was willing, even eager, to push the boundaries of what he called "longevity medicine."

Over the past six months, Shortt had already been visited by two of the team's starters—guard Kevin Donnalley and tackle Todd Steussie—both of whom he would later put on a regimen of human growth hormone and testosterone lozenges that he assured them would not be detected by the NFL. (A third, center Jeff Mitchell, would start visiting in May.) Now, he was going to do the same with Walls.

Once Walls introduced himself, he was led into a small office where he found Shortt waiting. After some doctor-patient small talk and a review of Walls's blood work, the physician launched into a description about what he wanted to prescribe.

"DHEA is a banned substance in this day and age," he began, referring to dehydroepiandrosterone, the naturally produced hormone that is a precursor of testosterone. As a result of the Dietary Supplement Health and Education Act of 1994, DHEA was making a fortune for companies that were eagerly—and hyperbolically—promoting it as a fountain-of-youth drug. The

NFL, however, considered it a steroid and so it remained on the banned list.

"I wouldn't use a huge dose," Shortt said. "I would use a small dose ... for you, a small dose like—I'm not talking a lot, I'm talking 10 milligrams, and for a guy your weight, that's like, *pfff*. But still, just to bring it up a little bit to help you deal with stress. And that should blow no whistles."

Walls, who didn't really know supplement lingo, was confused. "Is this, like, the testosterone patches?" he asked.

"No, no, no." Shortt answered. "This is DHEA. Because your DHEA levels are just at the bottom end of normal."

The next thing on Shortt's list was testosterone. The NFL monitored testosterone by measuring it against the presence of its chemical cousin, epitestosterone. Most people have equal amounts of both, yielding a 1:1 t/e ratio. But a small minority of individuals produces large amounts of testosterone naturally. Since the league can't punish players for their natural physiology, it sets its t/e ratio at 6:1 as an acknowledgment of the top end of the natural range. The flaw, of course, is that the rule allows players whose natural level is 1:1 the license to boost their testosterone levels within the legal limits of the policy.

Looking at the results of his blood work, Shortt told Walls: "For somebody like you, I can triple your testosterone levels without blowing any whistles.... Now, you can use patches. I don't know if there's anything in the patches that is testable. What I use for people is a cream, because there's nothing detectable in the cream ... and for you guys, what I'm looking for is non-detectable performance enhancement. And when we get to a minute—get to it in a minute, you can probably do well with a little bit of growth hormone. So that's—that's all I would do with you right there. Small amount of DHEA, not enough to blow any whistles, and testosterone."

Seeing Walls shift, Shortt added something to put him at ease. The NFL wasn't really interested in low-level doping, the doctor said. "It's in their best interest to level the playing field, but it's not in their interest to bust the whole damn team, you know. I mean, really, so they're not going to want to do that."

Walls nodded. There was no escaping the logic of what Shortt was saying: Only the greedy, or the really desperate, got caught.

FORT LAUDERDALE, FLORIDA

February 18, 2003

While Walls was debating whether to fill the prescriptions for testosterone and growth hormone that Dr. Shortt had given him[1] (he claims he never did), a South Florida medical examiner was reaching a grim conclusion about another performance enhancer: ephedra.

Early during a morning workout on Sunday, February 16, a pitching prospect for the Baltimore Orioles, Steve Bechler, started to feel dizzy and turned to a teammate to help prop him up. A decision was made to call paramedics and they found Bechler frighteningly overheated when they arrived. One would later say that the six-foot-two pitcher felt as if he had been pulled from a fire.

The EMTs stripped off the pitcher's jersey, wet him down with towels, and then carefully loaded him into an ambulance. By the time he arrived at North Ridge Medical Center, Bechler's temperature was 106 degrees. So many brain cells had burned up that his nervous system was in chaos, leaving his organs to fend for themselves. With one firewall after another falling to the consuming heat, his body was literally incinerating.

After a procedure to open his airway, Bechler seemed to be taking a turn for the better. His circulatory system had stabilized and his fever was down to a more manageable 102 degrees. But thanks to all the blood products and fluids that had been pumped into his system, he was almost unrecognizable. His pitching fingers,

---

1 Walls told the *Charlotte Observer* that he had never returned to Shortt after the February consultation.

once strong, were now grotesquely swollen. His face looked like he'd been in a bad bar fight. By mid-morning Monday, Bechler's body was shutting down. The first things to stop working were his lungs. His kidneys were next. Then shock set in, sending his blood pressure into a free-fall. At 10:10 a.m., Steve Bechler was pronounced dead.

When the medical examiner started investigating the cause, he discovered that a teammate had thrown a bottle of Xenadrine RFA-1, a weight-loss supplement containing ephedrine, into a clubhouse trash bin while Bechler lay burning up. The teammate later confided that Bechler was taking the pills—and had consumed three that day—because he had gained too much weight in the off-season. He remembered Bechler brooding about his weight and his conditioning and saying, "I messed up."

The NFL and International Olympic Committee had already banned ephedrine. But during negotiations over the last collective bargaining agreement, MLB's players had refused to add it to their list.

Baseball was still in its drug-fueled glory days.

WASHINGTON, D.C.

April 2003

For all his self-assurance, Terry Madden really did appreciate that something was wrong with the way his organization, the United States Anti-Doping Agency, was going about prosecuting supplement cases. He didn't want to chase after some pimply skateboarder who had taken a tainted multivitamin any more than the kid wanted to be chased. But the strict liability rules set down by the World Anti-Doping Agency were unforgiving.

If Madden's hands were tied when it came to prosecuting, he had a freer rein to pursue a political solution. Last fall, he had flown to Washington, D.C., to discuss his troubles with a high-powered lobbyist named Shawn Smeallie.

Over lunch near the Capitol, Madden complained that this supplement problem was getting out of control. Blue Cross Blue Shield had conducted a survey that showed a million teens nationwide had used supplements and an alarming 500,000 had experimented with steroids. Madden's agency was the catch basin for the ones who had flunked drug tests as a result.

"It's a public health issue," he said.

Smeallie took Madden's concerns to a New York Congressman, John Sweeney, who had introduced a bill calling for pre-market approval of ephedrine-based products. A few months later, the legislation wasn't going anywhere; all concerned knew that Orrin Hatch would turn the Senate into a dead end.

Still, Senator Hatch was more vulnerable on the issue than he had been a decade earlier, when he had muscled DSHEA through Congress. The death of Steve Bechler was causing a lot of finger pointing, and many of those fingers were pointed at the gentleman from Utah. A front-page article in the *Los Angeles Times* revealed how Hatch had helped block a previous FDA attempt to cut the daily dosage of ephedra by up to two thirds. It also showed how the senator's son recently opened a lobbying company that took in $30,000 from a supplement industry trade group. Given all the scrutiny, Hatch didn't protest the way he otherwise might when the FDA proposed putting more visible warning labels on ephedra products. It was a small but telling concession that showed that the attitude was turning on Capitol Hill.

SAN JOSE, CALIFORNIA
June 7, 2003

Publicly, Major League Baseball's players opposed drug testing. But in reality, a split had been forming. As early as 2000, at a meeting of the union's executive committee in Arizona, a pitcher declared that he was tired of giving up 500-foot home runs. Even everyday batters were getting irked at having to listen to sportswriters ask them why they couldn't keep up with the hitters whose slugging stats were through the roof. The union's chief, Don Fehr, had spent the better part of two years traveling from team to team, listening to their concerns and coming to the conclusion that something needed to be done.

At the same time, Commissioner Bud Selig, was taking a crash course in steroids. As Peter Keating reported in *ESPN The Magazine*, he met with a dozen team doctors in Milwaukee in 2001 and was told that the main medical problem in baseball was steroids. Alarmed, Selig instituted drug testing in the minor leagues, where there was no union to stand in his way.

The results from the 2001 season were worse than Selig had feared. Roughly 500 players—about 11 percent of those not on the MLB 40-man roster, tested positive. He didn't make the numbers public, but he did quietly tell Fehr that with some of those players headed to the majors, they had to do something.

The pressure on baseball to act quickly gained traction with two other disclosures: In May 2002, Jose Canseco, now out of the game and ready to speak about his steroid use, told Fox Sports Net that 85 percent of all players were probably juicing. The next month, the San Diego Padres third baseman, Ken Caminiti, a former National League MVP, admitted to *Sports Illustrated* that he had used them and put the number of his colleagues using at 50 percent—lower than Canseco's number, but still shocking. By midsummer, a *USA Today* poll of players showed that 79 percent of them favored some steroid testing.

The result was a compromise that only lawyers looking to avert a players' strike could love. The league would randomly test all its players once during the season, but it would be done anonymously. No one would ever know the results, and no one who tested positively needed to fear immediate punishment. The sole aim of the yearlong experiment was to see how deep the problem actually ran. If more than five percent of the players tested positive, it would trigger a more punitive testing system in 2003.

Victor Conte liked to claim that he had something called "Victor's knack." It had kicked in when he tried out for Tower of Power, and again when he lucked into defending C.J. Hunter in Sydney. Now that drug testing was a reality in baseball, it was kicking in again. During a barnstorming tour of Japan, Barry Bonds had bragged about BALCO to the Yankees' Jason Giambi, who soon after passed along his younger and less successful brother, Jeremy, an outfielder for the Boston Red Sox.

Bonds, meanwhile, introduced his trainer, Greg Anderson, to Gary Sheffield, the Atlanta Braves slugger, who was rehabbing his knees with Bonds's help. All became recipients of Patrick Arnold's Clear—dramatically increasing a circle that the nervous chemist worried was already too crowded. Those players, in turn, helped to bring in more players: Giants catcher Benito Santiago, former back-up catcher Bobby Estalella, and the ex-Giant outfielder Marvin Benard.

But baseball was the one sport where someone as high profile as Conte couldn't hide. An IRS agent named Jeff Novitzky happened to have been a member of the Bay Area health club where Bonds worked out with Anderson, and had become astonished by his size. According to an article by journalist Jonathan Littman in *Playboy*, Novitzky turned to a colleague during a court appearance one day and said, "That Bonds. He's a great athlete. You think he's on steroids?" When the fellow officer, a California Bureau of Narcotics Enforcement agent named Iran White, replied, "I think they're all on steroids," Novitzky demurred. "He's such an asshole to the press," White recalled him saying. "I'd sure like to prove it."

Novitzky lobbied his supervisors to green-light a probe of Bay Area Fitness, which had long been the subject of steroid dealing rumors, which would involve sending in White undercover. Beginning in early April 2003, White hung around the gym as a member, slowly gaining Anderson's confidence as he became a client. White did his job so well that Anderson offered to take him to Pac Bell Park to meet Bonds.

Unfortunately, Anderson also did his job extremely well. On this night, White was aroused from his sleep by a strange feeling and asked his wife to call paramedics. He could barely feel his limbs. When he arrived at San Jose's Kaiser Hospital, he was told he had a stroke caused by a clot that formed from a torn muscle. White figured he would be able to be back on his feet before too long. Then his body heaved and he suffered another massive episode. Suddenly, that left Novitzky's investigation as paralyzed as his undercover partner.

> LOS ANGELES
> *July 2003*

No matter what kind of a case is being investigated, it helps to have a witness who has an incentive to help. The same was true in Don Catlin's line of work. His discovery of Norbolethone raised more questions than it answered. Thankfully, help arrived in a small syringe that had been anonymously sent to Terry Madden's agency and then routed to Catlin for analysis.

Catlin turned to his front line of defense, the GC/MS machine that breaks steroid samples into tidy, recognizable elements. Once he ran the compound through the machine, he could see that he was dealing with a relative of his old friend, Norbolethone. Some clever chemist seemed to have added two double bonds to the basic molecule knowing that it would change the mechanics of how it broke down in Catlin's machine. Instead of dissolving into compounds that the GC/MS was programmed to detect, it would burst into pieces that the machine couldn't "see."

In other words, by slightly changing the molecular structure of Norbolethone, its creator had created an "invisible" steroid.

To make sure his theory was right, Catlin needed to make his own batch. It behaved exactly the way Catlin predicted. This new concoction was more than molecularly complex. It was a drug that held as many ambitions as structural surprises. For Victor Conte, it represented the gateway to powerful clients. For its creator, whom Catlin now was reasonably sure was Patrick Arnold, it represented a chance to strut across an industry where notoriety was its own reward. And for its users, it meant a chance to stay at the top for just a little while longer.

> BURBANK, CALIFORNIA
> *August 6, 2003*

Arnold Schwarzenegger was one of Jay Leno's favorite *Tonight Show* guests, an actor always up for a good gag, always prepared with material. And with California's Democratic governor, Gray Davis, facing a recall election, he had more material than usual.

No one actually expected Schwarzenegger to run against Davis. After all, Schwarzenegger was so friendly with Richard Riordan, the wealthy former mayor of Los Angeles who lived near him in Brentwood, that he had written out a statement endorsing Riordan for governor. The bit he had rehearsed for Leno was designed to lead into that statement.

Leno did his part. "Let me ask you about this," he said as Schwarzenegger got comfortable in his chair. "I know it's been weeks and people going back and forth, and it's taken you a while and you said you would come here tonight and tell us your decision. So what is your decision?"

The pre-arranged bit involved Arnold saying, "My decision is ..." just as a producer cued a censor's beep that obscured his words. But Leno couldn't simply leave it there. "We've joked about this," he continued, stepping out of his role as a comedian. "But seriously, what are you going to do? You said you were going to come here tonight and tell us. What are you going to do?"

Schwarzenegger wasn't ready to get serious, at least not yet. "My decision obviously is a very difficult decision to make," he said. "It was the most difficult decision to make in my entire life except the one in 1978 when I decided to get a bikini wax."

The laugh line was a way to sidestep the real issue: the intense scrutiny he would be under if he decided to run. Two years earlier, the *National Enquirer* had run a story called "Arnold's 7-Year Affair," complete with photos of Schwarzenegger and an ex-bodybuilder-cum-actress named Gigi Goyette, who was referred to as his mistress. The rigors of a campaign would surely cause the tabloid press to magnify the incident, and perhaps find new ones.

But Schwarzenegger had an ace in the hole, unknown to all but a very few. The supplement industry wasn't only guarding its interests in Congress, where Orrin Hatch remained its fervent ally. It was also on the lookout in statehouses across America. And few prizes were bigger than the governorship of California.

A major player in the industry was Schwarzenegger's old patron, Joe Weider, whose seven magazines, including *Muscle & Fitness*, derived most of their advertising from the supplement industry. When Weider decided to sell the stable, he found a suitor in American Media, an upstart company that had recently acquired a trifecta of supermarket tabloids—*National Enquirer*, *Globe*, and *Star*. Its CEO was a veteran magazine executive named David Pecker. During a private dinner with Weider, Pecker had brought up Schwarzenegger. According to Weider, Pecker believed the actor's links to the company were still vital to the magazines' interests.

"Joe, we've done enough on Arnold," Pecker confided, referring to the *Enquirer*'s coverage. "We're going to lay off of him. We're not going to pull up any dirt on him."

The previous month, Weider had arranged for Pecker to finally meet the star. Pecker told Schwarzenegger that he was prepared to pay a *minimum* of a $1 million a year for five years and one percent in the net print ad revenues for the Weider division of American Media, for him to hold the largely ceremonial title of executive editor at *Muscle & Fitness* and *Flex*. That was a potential payout of $13 million. But the most valuable part of the offer—the one Schwarzenegger intuitively understood—didn't involve what Pecker would do, but what he *wouldn't* do. Pecker didn't get into the details, but Schwarzenegger left with no doubt that Pecker would keep his tabloids from skewering him as a candidate.[2]

Now, appearing on the *Tonight Show*, Schwarzenegger was ready to bank on the check that Pecker had yet to write. Dispensing with the humor, he continued, "No, but I've decided that California is in a very disastrous situation right now.... And the man that is failing the people more than anyone is Gray Davis. He's failing them terribly. And this is why he needs to be recalled." Leno braced.

"This is why I am going to run for governor of the state."

BURLINGAME, CALIFORNIA
September 3, 2003

Victor Conte heard a commotion in the parking lot outside BALCO and ran to his front window just in time to see federal agents pouring out of seven black cars and race toward him.

Since his partner, Iran White, had had a stroke, Jeff Novitzky had resurrected his investigation of BALCO by rifling through the company's trash on Monday nights. On one of those runs, he had absentmindedly dumped the refuse he had been examining into the wrong dumpster. When the dumpster's owner found it, he angrily called Conte, who apologetically picked up the bag and returned it to BALCO. There, Conte found that smaller waste bags inside the large black one had been unsealed and rifled through. It was his first inkling that he was being watched.

---

2 "It's common sense," Schwarzenegger told writer Laurence Leamer, who was the first to chronicle the meeting in his 2005 book, *Fantastic: The Life of Arnold Schwarzenegger*. "Do you want to work with someone who you are attacking? You don't have to say anything. You don't have to be sleazy and make deals. It's human nature."

A cautious man might have laid low. But everything about Victor Conte's business plan rested on him maintaining a high profile. At the World Track Championships in Paris two weeks earlier, he sauntered around the athletes' warm-up area as if he owned it. His behavior drew a venomous reaction from his old business partner, Trevor Graham, who turned to a colleague as he watched Conte giving out supplements and said, "See that guy? He's going down."[3]

Now Novitzky was leading the raid through Conte's office while the window louvers clattered from the high winds caused by a helicopter hovering overhead. Novitzky told him that he wanted to talk and escorted Conte to the very same conference room in the rear where Project World Record had been hatched. The two men would recall what happened over the next two hours differently. Novitzky would claim that Conte confessed his whole operation in detail; Conte insists that he merely spoke generally. This much is clear, though: At two in the afternoon, Novitzky told Conte that he knew BALCO had a storage locker a half-mile away and wanted to see it.

For all that the government would make of this raid and the subsequent arrests, not much had changed since Dan Duchaine began his smuggling career by saying, "No one ever goes to jail for this." Of 941 federal busts for simple drug possession that reached the sentencing stage in 2003, the vast majority—698—were for marijuana. Steroids were so far down on the list that anyone who got caught using them was sure to get probation, not the maximum term of six months. Just as comforting to Conte, the laws defining a steroid were so cumbersome that the THG vials that awaited Novitzky in the storage locker couldn't even be considered a controlled substance.[4]

---

3 At the competition, one of Conte's prized clients, Kelli White, blazed her way to gold medals in the 100- and 200-meter dashes, only to subsequently test positive for the narcolepsy drug Modafinil. Conte started experimenting with it as a stimulant in early 2002, believing that drug testers weren't looking for it. More than a year later, they finally caught on.

4 A subsequent 42-count indictment did not include THG in the steroid distribution section. Instead, it was folded into a charge that accused him of misbranding drugs.

So Conte figured he might as well do what he was being asked. He climbed into the black car that was idling outside BALCO, and went on a short drive to the storage locker to show the IRS agent what he wanted to see.

17

STATE OF THE UNION

January 20, 2004 - November 4, 2004

WASHINGTON, D.C.

January 20, 2004

In his wildest dreams Terry Madden could not have imagined what the raid on BALCO would bring. The U.S. Attorney in San Francisco, Kevin Ryan, immediately empanelled a grand jury to take testimony from the lab's clients and the press went into a feeding frenzy. Madden did more than anyone to encourage it. After a small circle of reporters learned of Don Catlin's THG discovery, Madden held a phone conference to reveal, for the first time, the broad outlines of what was unfolding: how the syringe had been sent to USADA by a mysterious coach and then decoded by Catlin's lab, and how "several" track athletes were nabbed using it.

"What we have uncovered appears to be intentional doping of the worst sort," Madden said. "It's a conspiracy involving chemists, coaches, and certain athletes to defraud their competitors, and the American and world public who pay to attend sporting events."

The word conspiracy hung in the air. What did he mean? How

big a conspiracy? Madden stammered as reporters fired their questions. The feds had hoped to keep all of this quiet, but that was now clearly impossible. Madden had taken the story off the sports pages of every paper in America (except the *San Francisco Chronicle,* which had played it on A-1 two days earlier), and made it front-page news.

With the story out, reporters started stalking the federal courthouse in San Francisco in search of comments from major leaguers such as Barry Bonds and Jason Giambi, and Olympians like Tim Montgomery and Marion Jones, as they arrived for closed-door grand jury sessions.

Madden, of course, had no authority over pro sports, but he was desperately concerned about the BALCO-ites who were likely candidates for the Olympics. The Summer Games were only seven months away and he didn't have much time to bring cases. Unfortunately, Ryan was being noncommittal about cooperating, no doubt worried about Madden's penchant for holding impromptu press conferences.

Left to investigate on his own, Madden called Victor Conte's lawyers to arrange a face-to-face meeting at a hotel near the BALCO offices. It was two days before Christmas and he was hoping to have Conte's cooperation gift-wrapped. Unfortunately, Madden had a weak hand. He could offer to put in a good word with Ryan, but that was not exactly the ironclad guarantee that Conte's lawyers sought. So Madden left without anything.

His disappointment was acute, especially because he was drawing heat for another series of supplement cases. The latest poster boy for his critics' grievances was Kicker Vencill, a 24-year-old swimmer from Kentucky who had taken a multivitamin that turned out to be contaminated with 19-norandrosterone. Although the evidence suggested that Vencill was a victim, Madden took a hard line, aggressively pursuing a four-year ban. The young swimmer took the case to arbitration and lost, then appealed to the

Swiss-based Court for Arbitration in Sport, where he lost again. (Conceding that he did nothing intentional, the judges reduced his suspension to two years.) Vencill later successfully sued the supplement maker in state court and was awarded $578,635.

To Madden's detractors, the case was yet another sign that he was leading a principled but misguided war against innocent athletes. Pete Carey of the San Jose *Mercury News* reviewed the case files of 77 athletes punished by USADA and found that about half of them had tested positive for "substances commonly found in over-the-counter supplements and medicines."

The system Madden had set up four years earlier was at its breaking point. So, retreating to Colorado, he threw himself into his other crusade—convincing Congress to do something about the over-the-counter supplements that were humiliating USADA.

Now, early in the new year, Madden was back in Washington, taking what seemed like an endless series of meetings on the Hill. He had just gotten back to his hotel when his cell phone rang with a call from the White House Office of National Drug Control Policy.

"Watch the president's speech tonight," Michael Gottleib, the general counsel, told him. "There's going to be a little something in it for you."

After dinner, Madden settled in to hear an ex-owner of the Texas Rangers address the nation. More than two years after 9/11, George W. Bush's administration was still making terrorism its number-one priority and the President's opening words in his State of the Union speech showed the extent to which he was going to make it an issue in his upcoming re-election campaign, too.

"America this evening is a nation called to great responsibilities," he began. "And we are rising to meet them. As we gather tonight, hundreds of thousands of American service men and women are deployed across the world in the war on terror. By bringing hope to the oppressed, and delivering justice to the violent, they are making America more secure."

A half hour later, President Bush moved on to drug control. "One of the worst decisions our children can make is to gamble their lives and futures on drugs," he said. Generally, that would be enough for Madden, but Bush was about to give him the Christmas present he had missed in San Francisco.

"Athletics play such an important role in our society," the President continued. "But, unfortunately, some in professional sports are not setting much of an example. The use of performance-enhancing drugs like steroids in baseball, football, and other sports is dangerous, and it sends the wrong message—that there are shortcuts to accomplishment, and that performance is more important than character. So tonight I call on team owners, union representatives, coaches, and players to take the lead, to send the right signal, to get tough, and to get rid of steroids now."

Madden stared at his screen, speechless. The leader of the free world had just given him a prime-time dose of political clout.

Across the country, in San Diego, a father of two boys was driving home on Highway 15 when he heard the speech on his car radio.

It was Christmastime for Jack MacGregor, too.

SAN DIEGO

March 29, 2004

DEA agent Jack MacGregor [1] looked over the conference table surrounded by agents and felt a rush. The United States hadn't pursued a Mexican steroids case this big in 18 years. The last one came when Dennis Degan, the now-displaced FDA investigator, busted the Tijuana-based Laboratorios Milanos that was the source for Dan Duchaine. The yawning interval since then showed how far steroids had fallen off the government's radar.

This meeting showed just how much steroids had come back onto it. The U.S. Attorney General, John Ashcroft, had recently

---

1 Jack MacGregor is a fictional name chosen by the agent to protect his identity in ongoing investigations.

announced a 42-count indictment against the four figures at the heart of the BALCO case—Victor Conte and BALCO vice president James Valente, along with trainer Greg Anderson and track coach Remi Korchemny. That the case was grabbing national publicity escaped no one's notice.

MacGregor had become familiar with the Mexican drug trade while working on a previous case involving an animal painkiller called ketamine, which gained popularity in East Coast nightclubs as the rave drug Special K. The source for ketamine was a veterinarian named Jose Francisco Molina, who had just opened a state-of-the-art lab near Mexico City called Ttokkyo. (He had studied in Japan and loved the city.) Molina's partner was an ambitious 43-year-old businessman named Jorge Chevreuil Bravo, who had turned a veterinary supply store he had inherited from his father into a chain of 14 outlets along the U.S. border. After a year of using informants in Mexico, MacGregor had enough to arrest both men. When he learned that they would be traveling to Panama on September 17, 2002, he arranged take them into custody.

As he helped federal prosecutors ready the case for trial during 2003, MacGregor couldn't stop thinking about Ttokkyo's other top seller. While dealing ketamine, the two men had also helped to revolutionize the steroid trade by asking customers what they wanted. With that illicit bit of marketing, Molina started making high-dose blends of several different compounds that became so popular, American dealers were flying into Tijuana with hundreds of thousands of dollars in cash for Chevreuil Bravo.

Now that MacGregor had taken Ttokkyo down, others were rushing to fill the void. So the agent came up with the idea to target them all at once. Since steroids weren't part of the Ttokkyo case, the Mexican manufacturers would never see a steroid-based prosecution coming. At the very least, he'd have the element of surprise. Late in the fall, he drafted a proposal and gave it to a supervisor. "Can't you ever do anything simple?" he was asked.

By January, MacGregor had a green light from the DEA. But he still let out a whoop when he heard the President's State of the Union speech. The next day, his voicemail box was full of messages from headquarters, telling him that he would have everything he needed for the operation he was calling Gear Grinder.

Now, three months later, he was sharing the blueprint with a group of agents he had assembled from DEA offices in New York, Miami, Seattle, Philadelphia, and Lansing, Michigan—many of them veterans of Operation Ttokkyo. As they gathered around a large conference table in a downtown San Diego hotel, he flicked on a projector that displayed satellite photos of labs that he wanted to target, along with the men who owned them, and the steroids they produced.

"Ladies and gentlemen," he said. "We're here to eradicate Mexican steroids."

LONG BEACH, CALIFORNIA
April 8, 2004

With the BALCO case continuing to unfold, IRS agent Jeff Novitzky decided to attack baseball at its weakest point. The previous year, the league had negotiated a drug-testing agreement in which the results would remain confidential. Novitzky wanted to see whether any of the BALCO clients, particularly Barry Bonds, was on that list.

The fight to get those supposedly confidential records was nasty. In January, the San Francisco U.S. Attorney's office issued broad subpoenas to the two companies in charge—Comprehensive Drug Testing of Long Beach, California, which oversaw the program, and Quest Diagnostics of Teterboro, New Jersey, which collected the samples. After both balked at releasing the names of clients, another, narrower subpoena was issued, this one asking for the records of just 10 players with BALCO connections. Once again,

CDT went to court to quash the request, this time with the players' union rallying to its side.

That was scarcely enough to deter the feds. A day earlier, in a clever legal work-around, they had applied for a search warrant to seize what they could not get with a more appropriate subpoena. Now Novitzky and 11 other federal agents were walking into the offices of CDT to execute that search warrant. One of the office's directors was dumbstruck. Who did this six-foot-seven bald guy think he was?

While the director called the CDT's lawyer, asking what to do, a member of Novitzky's team came across a jackpot: a list that matched the names of all the players who had been drug tested to the numbers of their samples. Excited, Novitzky immediately faxed it to a waiting prosecutor in San Francisco. While he did this, the office director stormed out, visibly upset. When she came back, she opened a locked drawer and finally gave Novitzky what he wanted: a hard copy of the results for the 10 players he had requested.

Soon, even that extraordinary discovery wasn't enough for the agents. As the afternoon reached its midpoint, one of the office managers found a hard drive containing the records for the entire MLB program. When Novitzky's agents finally left CDT after five p.m., they had a disk with the records of the BALCO athletes they wanted, all the records of MLB, and 2,911 other files that contained secret information having to do with 13 other sports and businesses. MLB's union was officially on notice: The government was here to play hardball.

SACRAMENTO, CALIFORNIA
April 21, 2004

Jackie Speier wasn't about to be left behind on the steroid issue. The 54-year-old California lawmaker was raised in Burlingame, California, not far from BALCO. She subsequently became a supervisor in San Mateo, then became a state senator. One of Speier's biggest crusades was against Governor Gray Davis, whom she criticized for vetoing a bill in 2000 to ban ephedra products, when one of his campaign contributors was Metabolife, which made ephedra products. After the death of Orioles pitcher Steve Bechler, Davis finally signed the bill to make California the third state in the nation (after New York and Illinois) to ban ephedra.

Andro was next on Speier's hit list. The Secretary of Health and Human Services, Tommy Thompson, sent letters to 23 companies to warn them that they could be prosecuted if they kept selling Andro. But Speier felt the warning didn't go far enough. A mother of two, Speier was deeply troubled by the results of a University of Michigan study conducted in 2000 that claimed that 3.5 percent of 50,000 surveyed high school seniors admitted to using steroids at least once. Speier asked a Sacramento consulting group to do its own study and was even more alarmed when it reported that more than half of the high school athletes surveyed said that they knew of someone who had taken a performance-enhancing supplement or a steroid. The study had its obvious problems. Lumping a supplement like creatine together with steroids is like combining kidnapping and murder in the same statistic. Still, it gave her what she wanted: a pretext for two bills she was unveiling.

During a conference call with reporters, Speier announced that she wanted the most comprehensive anti-Andro law in the country. She said she wanted to ban the sale of Andro to minors, bar supplement companies from sponsoring school sports, require education among coaches, and, most controversially for a state drowning in budget deficits, she wanted spend roughly $80 million to mandate steroid testing among high schoolers.

The bill was aimed directly at the new man in the governor's mansion.

After announcing his candidacy on *The Tonight Show*, Arnold Schwarzenegger had shown remarkable deftness as a politician.

Days before the election, the *Los Angeles Times* released a campaign-shaking article that quoted six women as saying Schwarzenegger inappropriately groped them between 1975 and 2000. But the Terminator came back—Schwarzenegger went on a bus tour throughout the state that actually helped him pick up votes. After spending $22 million over two months, he had earned 48.6 percent of the nearly 8.5 million votes cast.

Yet for all his political dexterity, the governor seemed caught off-guard by Speier's move. Only a month earlier, he had been at his fitness expo in Columbus, meeting with supplement vendors and affirming his opposition to regulation. "I have very rarely seen the government do anything that was effective," the governor joked, doing his double duty as the executive editor of *Muscle & Fitness* and *Flex*.

Now Speier's bill had just put Schwarzenegger, the nation's leading steroid success story, between two rock-hard places.

COLORADO SPRINGS, COLORADO
June 23, 2004

Terry Madden wasted no time using the clout that the president had given him. With the Olympics in Athens nearing, he needed more than 9,000 documents that had been seized by the feds. Fortunately, he had a strong ally in Arizona Senator John McCain, who subpoenaed the documents from the U.S. Justice Department on his behalf. In a closed-door hearing, with Don Catlin at his side, Madden explained that time was running out. If they wanted to bring charges before the Olympics, they had to act immediately.

McCain ultimately gave Madden what he wanted: BALCO calendars with letters that denoted Insulin as I; Human growth hormone as G; EPO as E; THG, trenbolone, and Norbolethone as L; Clear as C; and a mix of testosterone and epitestosterone as either C, cream, L or lotion. Testosterone was C-Pure.

Still, they weren't enough for him to make a case that would stand up in court. What Madden needed was Victor Conte to interpret them. In a high-stakes meeting with prosecutors in San Jose on June 4, Conte's lawyers tried to work out a plea bargain with the feds that would include his testimony to USADA. But after three-and-a-half hours, the talks fell apart.

What happened next was controversial and, in Madden's view, necessary. Needing a way to make the documents fit the crime, he turned to his legal deputy, Travis Tygart, for an opinion. The memo he got back was precisely what was required. Its analysis said that USADA no longer needed to follow the standard of reasonable doubt in bringing cases. Instead, Tygart wrote, they could use a lower standard—one called "comfortable satisfaction" that had recently been adopted by the World Anti-Doping Agency.

Comfortable satisfaction? The lawyers who had to defend against the lower standard were incredulous. "I've never heard of it," said Cristina Arguedas, the exasperated lead attorney for Tim Montgomery. Marion Jones's lawyer, Joseph Burton, quipped that it sounded like a standard for buying sneakers, not for deciding an athlete's future.

But Madden was unbowed. What had he told USADA's board of directors that very first time he addressed them four years ago? "There are a lot of things you're going to be doing for the first time."

Well, here was yet another one. He green-lighted doping proceedings to be filed against Montgomery and three other BALCO clients (though not Marion Jones).

They were the first cases brought entirely on the basis of documents, *not a positive drug test*. On the most immediate level, it showed the world that USADA's days of going after 16-year-old fencers were over. Montgomery was the world's fastest man. The other three—Alvin Harrison, Chryste Gaines, and Michelle Collins—were all Olympic medalists.

But the significance of the cases was greater than even that. By bringing charges on the basis of documents alone, Madden had once again expanded the way he and his successors patrolled the sports landscape. He was no longer shackled by the catch-22 of doping: How do you catch a cheater if their drugs are designed to evade drug tests? The new rule allowed him to use any evidence that he could find.

If athletes around the country were worried about USADA's powers before, they had a whole new set of reasons to stay awake at night now.

SALT LAKE CITY

July 2004

Ten years had elapsed since Loren Israelsen helped pass the Dietary Supplement Health and Education Act. But despite all the money earned and all the campaign contributions made, the Salt Lake City attorney still thought about what he had told himself in the first hours after his industry's triumph: "We have to show that we deserve what we got. Otherwise, our critics are going to crucify us."

It had already begun with ephedra. Richard Durbin, the Democratic senator from Illinois, was so upset about the death of a 16-year-old high school football player in his district that he was pushing a measure that would force supplement companies to report adverse effects of their products to the FDA. Orrin Hatch, who had previously agreed to put warning labels on ephedra products, had already volunteered to work with Durbin on a bill. Now, the war was spilling into steroids.

At best, Israelsen saw Andro peddlers as distant cousins. At worst, he saw them as threats to his carefully constructed coalition. Either way, they were giving the industry a worse name than it already had on the Hill. At a hearing in the spring, baseball's union chief, Don Fehr, testified that he didn't see anything wrong with his players taking Andro, so long as it was legal. Never mind that it was banned in the Olympics and the NFL. Fehr didn't see why his players should be held to a different standard than the average American.

Senator McCain grew so angry at that suggestion that he practically spat out his reply. "Your failure to commit to addressing this issue straight on immediately will motivate this committee to search for legislative remedies," he said. "I don't know what they are. But I can tell you, and the players you represent, the status quo is not acceptable."

In fact, the status quo was already changing. The previous month, the House passed a bill to ban Andro and 26 other steroid precursors by a vote of 408-3. In the Senate, Hatch was working on a similar measure with Senator Biden, albeit with one key difference: The Senate bill exempted DHEA, the same drug that Dr. Shortt suggested to some of his sports patients, and which countless anti-aging clinics were dispensing.

Hatch was willing to clamp down hard on the first point, given all the indications that over-the-counter steroids were filtering down to high schools. But the anti-aging market was a thornier issue, particularly since it accounted for so much of Utah's $3 billion in annual supplement sales.

There was also plenty of reason to debate DHEA's effectiveness. In an interview with *The New England Journal of Medicine*, Dr. Elizabeth Barrett-Connor, department chair of family and preventive medicine at the University of California, San Diego, called it "the snake oil of the '90s." She went on to add, "It makes me very nervous that people are using a drug we don't know anything about. I won't recommend it." Nonetheless, anti-aging clinics were touting DHEA as another fountain of youth. The American Academy of Anti-Aging Medicine posted a February 2004 study on its Web site from the University of Wisconsin-

Madison to suggest that DHEA could help spur the production of brain cells in people as they aged.

The seemingly irreconcilable question was how Congress could police those who wanted to use it for performance enhancement, while also protecting the old. That question threatened to derail the bill until the DEA came riding to the rescue with a promise: If evidence mounted that DHEA was being used by teens more than by the elderly, the DEA would step in. While not a perfect solution, the pledge was enough for the Senate's biggest supplement skeptic, Dick Durbin, to go along with the compromise.

Now, the pieces were nearly in place. Israelsen's supplement coalition had banded with Terry Madden's sports world coalition to target a common enemy. It was a fragile marriage, but enough to signal that Congress was finally getting serious about ending the golden age of steroids.

LAS VEGAS

October 30, 2004

Judging from the booths in the exposition hall of the Mr. Olympia contest, the sports supplement industry was in a state of retrenchment. Many were empty. Those that remained were relying on sex, as barely clad women handed out samples like tarted-up department store dolls. On the far aisle near the back of the room, Patrick Arnold was hiding in plain sight. Ever since the BALCO raid, he had been a nervous wreck, wondering every day whether this would be the one when the feds came for him. Ironically, business was never better. It was such a good year that Arnold and his partner had bought themselves matching silver Lexuses. That's why he was mounting one last desperate attempt to stop Congress from enacting its Andro ban. With the help of his Long Island lawyer, Rick Collins, he began a group called the United Supplement Freedom Association and attempted to rally Steroid Nation. They sold shirts bearing the slogan "Your Body, Your Business," and urged customers to write their elected representatives.

But it was to no avail. Eight days earlier, Congress finally passed the Anabolic Steroid Control Act of 2004, putting 18 performance enhancers (including Arnold's own THG and Andro) on the controlled substances list.

By far the oddest presence at Mr. Olympia was Sylvester Stallone. After losing 44 pounds for a movie role, he had come up with an idea to launch his own supplement line and had chosen Patrick Arnold's younger brother, John, to be the company's CEO. In what could easily be construed as an epitaph for his brother's reign, John Arnold was all too willing to declare a new day at hand. "The (supplement) industry needs order," he told New York's *Daily News*. "There needs to be a high-profile leader. [Stallone] wants to be that leader."

In other words, things were so bad, an aging Rocky had to join the fight.

COLLEYVILLE, TEXAS
November 4, 2004

While IRS agent Jeff Novitzky was pursuing the world of professional sports, and USADA's Terry Madden was keeping an eye on the Olympics and the supplement industry, Lori Lewis, a five-foot-tall mother of two, was taking on Texas high school athletics.

Lewis lived in Colleyville, an upscale community of 20,000 located near the Dallas-Fort Worth Airport where the typical annual family income was $117,000 and the average house cost almost twice as much. One reason for the high property values was Colleyville Heritage High, a sharply designed, well-appointed school that reflected the community's ambitions. Just four years ago, the school had earned the 33rd spot on *Newsweek*'s list of top 100 public high schools. At the same time, its Panthers announced their arrival into the world of Friday Night Lights by going 10-2 and winning the Division 5A district championship.

Lori's son, Bryan, a skinny teen with a crooked smile, had spent the previous spring trying to decide whether he wanted to help the Panthers chase another title in 2004. As the quarterback of his junior varsity team, he had a leg up on the competition. But at nearly six feet and 160 pounds, everyone from his coach to his father—a former high school football star who was divorced from Lori, but who still lived close by—agreed that he needed to build strength.

One day in April, a fellow JV player confided to Bryan that he knew a senior who was dealing juice. The friends talked about the risks and rewards, and then agreed that they would experiment together. Bryan took $200 he had earned working at Applebee's and called the dealer to arrange a buy. In the driveway of his home on Crossgate Circle, Bryan nervously handed over the well-thumbed bills and in return got a 10 ml glass vial filled with hope.

He took the steroids with his teammate on a morning that he knew Lori wouldn't be home. The needle that went into his buttocks was supplied by a girl he knew. It was all very suburban, all very neat and tidy.

Unfortunately for Bryan, his closet wasn't. Several months later, Bryan had thought better of his little experiment. Maybe it was the back acne that felt so weird. Maybe it was the fact that the girl who had scored that first batch of needles wasn't up for another run. Or maybe it was the strange sensation he got after gaining 15 pounds of muscle that wasn't really his.

The reasons hardly mattered. Bryan decided to quit the football team and the steroids, and pursue baseball instead. It was all so casual that he had forgotten about the vial and three unused needles that lay inside a little white golf ball bag in his closet.

When Lori went through his dirty clothes six weeks later, she came across the golf bag. She absently moved it to one side when she heard something rattle inside and discovered Bryan's discarded stash. As Lewis would later tell magazine writer Craig Offman, her mind left her body. She reached for a phone to call the local Walgreen's and read a pharmacist what was printed on the vial: Nandrolone deaconate. After being told that it was an anabolic steroid, her fear melted to white-hot anger and she jumped in her Lincoln Navigator to drag Bryan home.

"Where did you get these?" she demanded through tears. Bryan had a hard time understanding her tone, especially since he had already made his own decision to reject the muscle-building drug.

"Mom, half the team is on it," he replied. That wasn't enough for Lewis, who wanted to know where he had got it. Bryan mentioned the name of the friend with whom he had purchased the drugs, but not the dealer.

The next day, Lewis called the school to reveal what she had found. Notes kept by the assistant principal, and reviewed by Offman, would cast her as an insistent, occasionally "hysterical" woman. But she was specific about Bryan and his friend. Three hours after her call, the assistant principal phoned again to say he had spoken with the Panthers coach, Chris Cunningham, and the coach insisted that there was no problem with steroids at Colleyville Heritage High.

If it had been Jeff Novitzky handling the investigation, search warrants would have been flying. If it had been Terry Madden, doorbells would have been ringing at all hours of the night. But this was high school sports. Who did Lori Lewis have to approach?

She chose a reporter from the community weekly, *The Colleyville Courier*. From a wing-backed chair in her living room, Lewis started telling her story to Scott Price. As she spoke, Lewis wasn't sure what kind of wellspring she was tapping. Would she get a vote of sympathy from the other moms, a you-go-girl pat on the back? She surely didn't expect what would result from the October 1 story that began:

A Colleyville mother called The Courier *because she found syringes and anabolic steroids in the room of her son, a local high school student. The woman wanted to remain anonymous to protect her son from reprisals. The woman said she asked her son where he got the steroids, and her son told her that he got the drugs from other students in his school.*

The month since was a nightmare. Though her name had been withheld by *The Courier*, the guessing game of "who snitched?" spread like wildfire through Colleyville Heritage High. A former player, now in another school, came under so much suspicion for being the leaker that he got a text message on his cell phone that said, "Watch your back, bitch."

And Bryan Lewis wasn't the only one feeling the heat. Price was getting hate mail at the offices of *The Courier*. A former pitcher for the Texas Rangers, whose son was attending Colleyville Heritage High, wrote to the reporter, asking why the hell he was stirring up so much trouble.

It was almost like a small-town horror movie, in which everyone was keeping a secret that an outsider had just stumbled onto. Except Lori Lewis wasn't an outsider. This was her town.

At least, it used to be her town.

It didn't feel that way anymore. With the furor still swirling, and the bigger *Dallas Morning News* starting to investigate, the Panthers were a team torn apart. As a former player would tell Offman, any alert observer could see the strange goings-on in the Panthers' locker room. There were the unusual rashes of back acne, spontaneous bouts of crying, suspicious muscle injuries. But when Coach Cunningham asked his players if they were using, they simply denied it.

Going into the season's final game against archrival Grapevine, an atmosphere that was supposed to be charged with pride was heavy with humiliation instead. One Grapevine fan ridiculed the Panthers fight slogan, "Bustin' Loose," by holding up a sign that read, "CHHS ain't bustin' loose—they takin' juice." The Panthers were so dispirited in the second half that they totaled just 85 yards in a 28-17 drubbing.

With the season now done, Lewis held out hope that the air could finally be cleared. But Cunningham, a Christian who coached values, was in a combative mood when he sat down with reporters for the *Morning News*. Speaking about Lewis, whose name was still not publicly known, he said, "This whole thing could have been made up about her son. This lady is a liar. There's nobody in my program who's on steroids. If there was, I'd be the first one to do something about it. You've got a crazy mom who's looking for someone to blame for her problem."

Shortly after that interview, a player on the team who looked up to Cunningham knocked on his office door and said, "Coach, can I talk to you?" Once he seated himself, he said what no one else in Colleyville had been willing to admit: The players were lying to him, not Lori Lewis.

By mid-December, nine players would step forward to admit what they had done—the most ever to confess in a high school steroids case. Coach Cunningham, however, didn't call the police to report the crime—he called the parents. Four sets confessed that they knew what their sons were doing, according to the internal school notes reviewed by Offman. A fifth father admitted he had done steroids in college and knew his son was using, too.

For all the attention that was being paid to BALCO, a single suburban mother in Texas had shown the real depth of steroid use in America.

18

THIS IS WAR

January 2005 - December 14, 2005

Jack MacGregor might never have heard of Don Catlin if his brother hadn't read the article in *Playboy* mentioning the doctor's involvement in the BALCO case. After learning about the work Catlin was doing, MacGregor called to request a meeting.

As they sat in a conference room at the UCLA analysis lab, MacGregor expanded on what he had told his fellow DEA agents 10 months earlier in San Diego. In Mexico, the steroid trade was perfectly legal. But in order to bring an indictment in United States against the men who were producing them, MacGregor had to prove three things: The first was that the high-dose brands being produced in Mexico were explicitly designed for humans, not animals. Second, that those doing the producing knew for what purpose they were being used. And finally, that they also knew the drugs were bound for the United States. As the agent would later say, "The hurdle was *specific intent.*"

Proving that the lab owners knew they were breaking American law required more investigative resources than MacGregor had used to help indict Jose Francisco Molina and Ttokkyo. Beginning in the early winter, he and a partner who specialized in prescription drugs started scrutinizing each of the DEA's eight analysis labs for all the steroids that had been seized in 2003. The results shocked him: $56 million in steroid sales came from eight different companies. Seven out of every 10 sales came from the same three Mexico City labs. And those labs were all registered to a group that included a California-trained veterinarian named Alberto Saltiel-Cohen.

Saltiel-Cohen didn't own expensive cars or cigarette boats—none of the usual big-time drug dealer perks. Rather, he lived the life of a pharmaceutical executive, well-to-do, but low-key. His company, Denkall, was ostensibly in the veterinary medicine business. But in the late 1990s, he had started competing with Molina's Ttokkyo on the steroid front by making blends with compounds that weren't easily available in America. To help market them, two of his companies, Quality Vet and Animal Power, launched Web sites with cute animals on their Web pages that hid their real intent.

Having one group responsible for so much traffic brought MacGregor's case into sharp relief, but it also exposed the problems he would have. In a traditional drug case, agents made undercover buys, arrested the dealers, and tried to flip them so they could work their way to the top of the pyramid. But the economics of steroids conspired against that. The sentencing law for Schedule III drugs required that a dealer had to sell 40,000 "dosage units" to qualify for a maximum sentence of five years. That would have meant spending hundreds of thousands of dollars to arrest just one person. There was no way that the DEA could finance that.

Instead, MacGregor started from the bottom, targeting the distributors who bought in bulk from Saltiel-Cohen. Since a grand jury had been empanelled in July 2004, he had been using informants to place orders on DEA-issued BlackBerries, then saving their e-mails as proof that the distributors knew they were selling animal steroids to humans.

If he ever got to the top of the pyramid, MacGregor would need an expert to testify that the steroids being sold were the same ones commonly used by athletes. That's where Catlin came in. It was the second time in as many years that a federal investigator was asking for his help, and Catlin said he would do all he could.

> CHICAGO
> *January 2005*

While the DEA was waging the biggest attack on steroids in two decades, there were growing signs that Americans were becoming increasingly ambivalent about this branch of the war on drugs, and that they had real questions about whether it was even sustainable.

There was perhaps no greater symbol of the country's skepticism than a former steroid critic named Bob Goldman. In the 1980s, Goldman had gained fame for his trilogy of books—*Death in the Locker Room: Steroids & Sports*; *Death in the Locker Room: Steroids, Cocaine & Sports*; and *Death in the Locker Room II: Drugs & Sports*. The opening line of the first one showed his uncompromising attitude: "The time is ripe. We need the truth."

But as he started getting older, Goldman replaced his righteous fire with an appreciation for the anti-aging industry. He formed a group called the American Academy of Anti-Aging Medicine (A4M) and started putting on increasingly popular conventions.[1] The World Congress on Anti-Aging Medicine that he had just held in Chicago drew thousands of attendees and scores of vendors. Like the life extensionists who had come before them, Goldman's organization shared a common conviction: that aging is a form of disease and

---

1 As the *Los Angeles Times* pointed out in July 2006, Goldman also stretched his credentials while doing it. Though he earned a medical degree at Central America Health Sciences University in Belize, it was not recognized by the state of Illinois, where the A4M is based, causing officials there to fine Goldman $5,000 for using MD beside his name.

managing a patient's hormone levels is a medically legitimate way to slow it down.

The FDA, of course, disagreed. It did not consider aging a legitimate medical condition and didn't endorse hormone therapies to "cure" it. But A4M's press materials boasted that it had trained 30,000 practitioners, and none of them seemed terribly concerned with the FDA's oversight. One reason was that the agency seemed half-hearted about enforcing those rules. In response to a Freedom of Information Act request, the agency acknowledged that out of 55 criminal cases that were opened into steroid-related infractions in 2005, the worst penalty that it had meted out was a warning letter.

None of this suggested that Jack MacGregor's efforts in Operation Gear Grinder were misguided. One of the main things motivating MacGregor was a photo of Taylor Hooton he kept in his DEA office cubicle. After the 17-year-old Texas pitcher died by hanging himself in July 2003, his father created a foundation to warn others about steroids.

MacGregor saw Gear Grinder as an extension of Hooton's efforts to keep steroids away from kids. But what about adults? Just as tobacco or alcohol is legal for those who can make adult choices, why shouldn't steroids be? That was the question that Bob Goldman was posing.

And, judging from his success, he was doing a hell of a job.

SHENZHEN, CHINA
February 2, 2005

Bruce Kneller sped down a rural road in a taxi with views of Hunan Province outside his window and his wife at his side. It was his fourth trip to Mainland China in the last 18 months, and he was getting as comfortable navigating the countryside as he was navigating China's pharmaceutical industry.

Just as rushing water inevitably finds holes in cement, Kneller was having an easy time finding his way around the 2004 Anabolic Steroid Control Act. The law specifically banned 42 compounds, but by changing a few molecules in a steroid called Oral-Turinabol—an old favorite of East Germany's Olympic doping machine in the '70s and '80s—he was able to produce a product called Halodrol.

As Kneller would say later in an interview, "There was a lot of good German data on Oral-Turinabol and I spent a lot of time online and in medical libraries reading it. What I liked about it was that it was a whole lot less toxic than anything else being sold as a pro-hormone."

All he needed was a pharmaceutical company that could modify Oral-Turinabol on a large scale. And that was why he was in China.

If Mexico was the biggest source of steroids to the United States, China was the supplier to the world. The country produced much of them for legitimate drug resellers who then supplied hospitals and doctors. But much of what China produced also found its way into a murky middle ground. Kneller, like most Americans, had been dealing with brokers to get what he needed. But he knew that he could make more, and guarantee better quality, if he cut out the middlemen and sourced it out on his own.

"China is a giant factory," he would say. "People will make whatever you want. The same thing is true in Eastern Europe, but the Chinese are better and faster and they do it with less hassle."

Kneller also enjoyed the people he was meeting. If he made a demand that a host of theirs was uncomfortable with, he would be told that "it was inconvenient"—not that it couldn't be done. When one pharmaceutical executive had to cancel an appointment because his father had died that morning, he sent Kneller a basket of flowers with a kind note, stunning the American, who had been about to do the same thing himself.

As he crisscrossed the country, Kneller became conversant in the Chinese art of *guanxiwang*, or networking. Not every factory he visited was worth a return. One was little more than a corrugated hut where stone-faced laborers mixed powders in dirty vats over an open flame; there was almost no way to tell what was in those containers, but at least a half dozen of the Chinese plants were thoroughly modern, with the latest in German and American technology.

What Kneller loved most, however, was the beautiful young translator whom he had met on his first visit, and proposed to soon after. Now, two days before the Chinese New Year, he was heading to be with her parents in the village of Shaodong.

It was nearly midnight—and the two had been on the road for hours when their driver briefly closed his eyes from exhaustion. As the taxi veered into a guardrail, the shocked driver swung the wheel to the right, causing the car to swerve wildly in the opposite direction. Kneller's arm was crushed trying to keep his wife safe as the taxi slid off an embankment and tumbled down a ravine, side over side. When it finally stopped, Kneller smelled smoke and realized that the undercarriage had caught fire. The onetime nurse maneuvered his leg so that he could kick the door open and dragged his wife to safety, just in time to crawl clear of an explosion. Luckily, a passing bus shone its lights into the rice paddies and spotted them. After an ambulance was summoned, Kneller awoke in a nearby hospital, listening to a doctor talk excitedly.

"What is he saying?" Kneller asked his wife.

"He's saying that he wants to amputate your arm," she replied.

Kneller bolted upright.

"Tell him that we're getting the hell out of here," he said.

WASHINGTON, D.C.

March 15, 2005

Representative Tom Davis eased into the Capital Grille, located a few blocks from his office in the Rayburn House Office Building, and greeted his dinner companion, Jose Canseco. In three days, Davis, a rising star in the House Republican leadership, was going to call Canseco and five other players to testify before his Government Reform Committee on steroids in baseball. He reportedly had tried to call Attorney General Alberto Gonzales to get immunity for the retired slugger, but a last-minute deal couldn't be worked out. So Davis was having dinner with Canseco to find out what he would be willing to say on the record.

A month earlier, on February 13, Canseco had appeared on *60 Minutes* to promote a tell-all book called *Juiced*. With Mike Wallace raising a skeptical eyebrow, Canseco admitted, "I tried to do everything possible to become the best player in the world. Do I believe steroids and growth hormones helped me achieve that? Yes. Were there a lot of other players doing it that I had to compete against? Yes." Then he looked Wallace in the eye and said that he had personally injected Mark McGwire.

Canseco's appearance and Commissioner Bud Selig's refusal to look into the allegations made Representative Henry Waxman, the committee's ranking Democrat, write to Davis to say that they needed more answers. Davis knew the move wouldn't make him popular with his friends in baseball—such as the owner of the Baltimore Orioles, Peter Angelos. Still, he was stunned by the chilly reaction he received when he announced that the committee was seeking the testimony of Selig and seven players—Canseco, McGwire, Jason Giambi,[2] Rafael Palmeiro, Curt Schilling, Sammy Sosa, and Frank Thomas.

Selig refused to meet Davis. Instead, in a political slight that didn't go unnoticed, he dispatched a paid lobbyist to Capitol Hill. (He later testified before the Committee.) The league also waited until the last minute to turn over a copy of a new drug-testing policy that had just been negotiated, forcing Davis's staff to stay up

---

2 Giambi would later be excused after union lawyers protested that he wouldn't be able to talk about his secret grand jury testimony.

all hours to digest it.[3]

The players weren't much more cooperative. Palmeiro announced that he had to attend his wife's birthday on the day of the hearings. McGwire sent word that he "respectfully declined" to attend. Davis finally had to issue subpoenas to show that he was serious.

Once it was clear there was no way out for the players, McGwire's attorney called Davis to ask for a private meeting. On the day before the hearings, a suited McGwire showed up to the Rayburn Office Building and was escorted into an empty hearing room.

When Davis walked in, he was struck by the size of the retired slugger: McGwire seemed half as large as Davis remembered. More than a year later, Davis would recall, "We spent a long time talking. I came away with the impression that he wasn't going to lie about what he did [in baseball] before Congress."

Canseco told Davis the same thing. As they dug into their steaks, the former Bash Brother was forthcoming about himself. "Look, the Rangers invested millions in me," he told the congressman. "They knew everything about me. Who I'm screwing, where I'm sleeping. You don't think they knew what I was putting into my body, what all of us were doing?"

But when it came to McGwire, he warned that the slugger wouldn't be as open. "Mark and I weren't best friends, but I know him. He can't, he won't, lie about what he did. But he won't talk about it either."

---

3 After more than five percent of major league players tested positive for steroids in 2003, a permanent drug testing policy was finally instituted. In the summer of 2004, the owners cut a deal with the players' union to give anyone who flunked a test for the first time private counseling and a possible ban if they flunked again. At the end of the year, MLB announced that fewer than two percent of players tested positive. But as the winter wore on, a torrent of revelations came out that cast doubt on those numbers. On December 2, the *San Francisco Chronicle* reported that in testimony before a federal grand jury, Yankee Jason Giambi admitted using the Clear and the cream from BALCO. A few days later, *ESPN The Magazine* published a detailed interview with Victor Conte in which he said that the current state of drug testing was so weak that cheating was "like taking candy from a baby." With several Congressmen openly calling for a federal takeover of drug testing in pro sports, the players voted to give union chief Donald Fehr the power to negotiate new penalties. On January 20, a deal was struck in which every player would be randomly tested once a season and given a 10-game ban for a first offense.

And three days later, he didn't.

The hearing was elaborately choreographed. The five witnesses (Thomas was interviewed via satellite) were kept in separate rooms with the televisions tuned to C-Span, so they could watch how the stage was being set for their testimony. And members were told that the players wouldn't be signing autographs, so they shouldn't bother to ask. In one small concession to his witnesses, Davis agreed to swear them in individually, rather than in unison, as is often the custom. The reason: Sosa, McGwire, Schilling, and Palmeiro[4] so despised Canseco, they refused to take the same oath as him.

Canseco wasn't exactly the witness Davis had hoped for. Without immunity, his most meaningful testimony came from the incredulous looks that he shot at the others while they answered their questions. "From what I'm hearing … I was the only individual in Major League Baseball to use steroids," he said at one point. "That's hard to believe."

Fairly or not, the afternoon centered on McGwire. Had he chosen to admit to steroid use, he might have been remembered as the heroic figure he hoped to be. He might have been seen as Representative Davis saw him: "As a decent guy who got caught up in something everyone else was doing."

But America wasn't privy to his closed-door disclosures. All they saw was a former baseball hero who refused to talk about a past that was quickly unraveling. When pressed about whether he was invoking his Fifth Amendment right against self-incrimination, McGwire famously insisted, "I'm not here to talk about the past."

---

4 When Palmeiro was named as a steroid user by Canseco—his former neighbor in Colleyville, Texas—he angrily waved a finger at Representative Davis and denied it. But six weeks after the hearing, Palmeiro failed a random drug test that found stanozolol in his system. The finding wasn't announced until August 1, at which time Davis's committee launched a perjury investigation. The 46-page final report concluded that charges weren't warranted against Palmeiro because the "detection window for stanozolol [is] as long as four weeks, [and] the Committee is unable to conclude that [he] took—either purposefully or inadvertently—the stanozolol that resulted in his positive test result before March 17, 2005, the date of his congressional testimony." But Victor Conte told this author that he had experiences with clients who took stanozolol and had it show up in drug tests six or seven weeks later. That at least would leave open the possibility that Palmeiro could have had it in his system at the time of his testimony.

And when North Carolina Republican Patrick T. McHenry asked him whether he thought using steroids was cheating, McGwire tried to sum up all the ambiguity he felt, and all the ambiguity he hoped America felt.

"That's not up to me to determine," he said simply.

> SAN FRANCISCO
> *July 15, 2005*

As the most famous steroid dealer in America, Victor Conte vowed that he was going to give the sports world a trial for the ages. But after spending 17 months under indictment, he was worn down.

There was a time, early on, when Conte was so sure that he held the upper hand in his dealing with prosecutors in the BALCO case that he came clean (with this writer) in the December 20, 2004, edition of *ESPN The Magazine*. In the article, he claimed to have witnessed Marion Jones use human growth hormone in an Embassy Suites hotel in Covina, California, on April 21, 2001.

"We'd had a lot of success since the previous August," he wrote, "after I'd arranged for her to receive various performance enhancers, including The Clear ... She was on all of it at the 2000 Games in Sydney, when she won three gold medals and two bronzes. I tell you this knowing Marion passed a lie detector test saying it's not true. All that shows me is lie detectors don't work." (These statements became part of the $25 million defamation suit Jones filed against Conte in December 2004, which was later settled out of court.)

All the money that Conte was making from his infamy, however, didn't make up for the unrelenting stress. He felt responsible for dragging his partner, Jim Valente, into this mess, along with the Ukrainian coach Remi Korchemny and trainer Greg Anderson, which is, in part, why he was agreeing to come forward at the Phillip Burton Federal Building to plead guilty.

While Kevin Ryan, the U.S. Attorney in San Francisco, attempted to paint Conte's pleas as a victory in the war on drugs, the denouement actually seemed to be further evidence of the nation's steroid schizophrenia.

Even if the BALCO men had been convicted of all 42 counts in the indictment, they couldn't have gone away for more than a year. So, not only did Ryan agree to drop all but two counts of the indictment that had been announced with such fanfare, but he also allowed a deal in which Conte would plead to the two felony counts of steroid distribution and money laundering and serve four months in federal prison followed by four months home confinement. (Anderson would plead guilty to the same two felony counts and serve three months and three months home confinement; Valente would plead to one felony count of distribution and receive probation; and Korchemny would later plead to one misdemeanor count of distributing modofinil and would also get probation.) All without providing any cooperation to the government.

By the second anniversary of the federal raid on BALCO, the case seemed to have less to do with sports, and more to do with a war whose aims were becoming increasingly cloudy. In fact, the lasting legacy of BALCO would have nothing to do with steroids, but with troubling offshoots of the case.

The U.S. Attorney's Office in Los Angeles eventually launched an investigation into the leaking of grand jury testimony, threatening two *San Francisco Chronicle* reporters with prison time if they didn't reveal their source.[5]

To prevent IRS agent Jeff Novitzky from using the fruits of his raid on baseball's drug-testing labs, the players' association would file three separate legal challenges that made their way to the 9th Circuit Court of Appeals. While two judges would rule

---

5 The issue was rendered moot when Troy Ellerman, an attorney who represented BALCO defendant James Valente, admitted in federal court that he let *Chronicle* reporter Mark Fainaru-Wada read secret grand jury documents. (In February 2007, he pleaded guilty to contempt of court, obstruction of justice, and making a false declaration.)

that Novitzky's hardball tactics were allowable, a third judge would accuse him and his superiors of all but tearing up the 4th Amendment by seizing computer hard drives without probable cause or a valid search warrant.

Finally, the government would force Greg Anderson back to jail once he had served his three-month sentence for refusing to testify in a grand jury about his former client Barry Bonds, slowly turning Anderson into a martyr for the steroid era of baseball.

TRIESTE, ITALY
July 20, 2005

From *Stars and Stripes:*

By Sandra Jontz

Italian police have busted an international drug ring that had been sending steroids and performance-enhancing drugs to U.S. soldiers in Iraq who, Italian investigators say, were ordering them via the Internet.

But for unknown reasons—possibly security precautions—the packages and envelopes of drugs were not reaching some of the troops, said Mario Bo, head of the criminal division for the Trieste, Italy, police department.

Instead, the drug-filled parcels addressed to U.S. troops in Iraq were being returned to an Italian post office in Trieste, and because dealers had not included a return address, they piled up, prompting postal officials to call police, Bo said.

As of Tuesday, no U.S. military officials had approached Italian officials for the names of prospective buyers in Iraq, Bo said.

Officials at the U.S. military command in Iraq said Tuesday that they were looking into the issue but could not provide more details by deadline.

U.S. troops were not the only "clients" among the long list of buyers from France, Great Britain, Belgium, Puerto Rico, the United States and Canada, Bo said....

"We do not have this problem in Deuce Four," Lt. Col. Erik Kurilla, commander for 1st Battalion, 24th Infantry Regiment, now serving in Mosul, said in an e-mail. "We do 100 percent health and welfare checks often, basically lock down a unit and go through everything looking for anything illegal. We have never found drugs or steroids.

"I have heard of only a few cases of drugs in other battalions supplied by interpreters, but this has never surfaced in Deuce Four. Our mail clerk also handles every package that arrives in the battalion and he has not seen strange European addresses either."

Similar responses came from troops serving in Baghdad and Marines in Fallujah....

The packages contain names and ranks of U.S. service members who presumably ordered the steroids via the Internet and prepaid using credit cards, Bo said. He declined to provide the Internet address that was selling the drugs.

While names of troops serving in Iraq can be found in the public domain—including on Web sites where troops can ask for specific care packages from strangers —there would be no money to be made by drug dealers randomly mailing steroids to troops, Bo said.

Drug testing in a combat zone is determined by each of the service's surgeon generals' offices, U.S. military officials said.

LA JOLLA, CALIFORNIA
December 14, 2005

Jack MacGregor thumbed the photo taped to his dashboard and scanned nine other DEA cars that had taken up positions around the posh Empress Hotel. As shoppers began filling the sidewalks, the agent kept his eye on the hotel lobby for the man in the photo, Alberto Saltiel-Cohen.

Over the past year, MacGregor had been closely following the steroid debate and had watched the Congressional hearings like everyone else. He kept coming back to what was said by Donald Hooton, the heartbroken father who believed that steroids had driven his son to suicide: "Players that are guilty of taking steroids are not only cheaters. You are cowards."

Every time that MacGregor thought of Saltiel-Cohen, he thought of Taylor Hooton, mainly because the vial of steroids that Hooton used—Deca QV 300—had been made by Saltiel-Cohen's company, Quality Vet.

Thanks to the informants he had working over the border, MacGregor was able to learn a lot about Saltiel-Cohen's Mexico City operation, and how he had used it to insulate himself. Distributors who had set up shop in tourist-friendly towns like Cancún, Nuevo Laredo, and Tijuana did all the heavy lifting. They arranged for sales of the products via e-mail or their Web sites, then had them smuggled to buyers in the United States. Saltiel-Cohen and his partners were then safely removed from the end of the line—the American dealers who sold the products until they ended up in high school locker rooms or in some middle-aged desk jockey eager to buff up.

In the end, Saltiel-Cohen was caught in an old-fashioned sting operation: MacGregor invented a phantom millionaire who was supposedly eager to buy into the steroid market. The DEA then created a bogus Web site—bio-power-meds.com—to show how serious he really was.

By September 16, the grand jury in San Diego had enough evidence to indict Saltiel-Cohen along with 22 others. But the U.S. Attorney's Office in San Diego made sure that the case file was sealed. If Saltiel-Cohen and the others learned that they had been indicted while still in Mexico, they would never cross the border. (Mexico rarely extradited its citizens.) So MacGregor had to wait for Saltiel-Cohen to travel on his own.

The three months since the indictment had been handed down were excruciatingly long. But now, finally, it was showtime. MacGregor's informants had convinced Saltiel-Cohen and four partners to travel north for a meeting with their fictitious steroid mogul. They were under the impression that they were going to strike a huge deal. They were wrong.

Once MacGregor spied the man in blue jeans and a leather jacket coming out of the hotel, he radioed to his men. "Arrest him."

Saltiel-Cohen wasn't known to carry any weapons, and he didn't have a bodyguard with him. Still, four agents quietly surrounded the Mexican businessman, flashed their badges, and told him that he was now in the custody of the U.S. Department of Justice. Similar arrests were made elsewhere in San Diego and Laredo, Texas.

Later that day, with five people under arrest (nine would eventually be charged), MacGregor called Donald Hooton to ask if he would like to fly to the press conference being held the next day in San Diego. Hooton, a marketing executive for Hewlett-Packard, jumped at the chance.

In an interview about the case a year later, MacGregor would talk openly about his Christian faith, more than once calling his pursuit of the Mexican steroid dealers, and Saltiel-Cohen in particular, "a cause." Hooton, he believed, was an important symbol for that cause: a man whose unimaginable loss showed parents the perils of ignoring their children. MacGregor was moved to be able to partly avenge that loss.

In law enforcement terms, it was the case of a lifetime, as evidenced by the gauntlet of hands that were waiting to shake Jack MacGregor's when he returned to the DEA's offices.

But in public policy terms, his success opened up a new set of issues.

The Mexican steroid trade wasn't going to die. As *Sports Illustrated* writers George Dohrmann and Luis Fernando Llosa pointed out in an article about the case, the steroid industry was simply going to be driven further underground, where the steroids sold were more likely to be counterfeit or toxic.

That wasn't an excuse for letting Saltiel-Cohen flaunt American law, but it did prove that steroids were no different than any other drug the DEA tried to control.[6] As a senior law enforcement official not involved with Operation Gear Grinder put it: "The DEA isn't going to be able to change behavior with steroids, any more than it has with cocaine or marijuana. The demand will always be there unless there's education, too."

---

6 Saltiel-Cohen's three companies eventually pleaded guilty to conspiracy to distribute controlled substances and aiding and abetting international monetary transactions and agreed to forfeit $1.4 million.

19

A VICIOUS CYCLE

February 17, 2006 - November 22, 2006

CANTON, MASSACHUSETTS

February 17, 2006

The Chinese doctor who tried to amputate Bruce Kneller's arm was the least of his problems. When he returned to the United States, there was no shortage of people who were waiting on line to cut him off at the legs.

One of them was Jack MacGregor, who along with the Operation Gear Grinder task force, had stumbled onto him. It started with a tip about an underground company called Red Star Laboratories and an e-mail address. After agents sent an e-mail to the account posing as a customer, they received a price list and even a special Christmas holiday brochure. The payment arrangements were specific: Buyers had to send money wrapped in tinfoil to one of several P.O. boxes that had been rented around San Diego with homespun names like Pewter & Porcelains. Eventually, the agents were able to track the addresses back to Kneller. After an associate picked up the cash, Kneller fulfilled the orders by mailing them from his local post office under the name "Mr. B's Internet eBay Auctions."

Three days earlier, on Valentine's Day, Kneller had driven eight miles from his home to the post office with 15 packages. He was calm and relaxed, smiling at the clerks as he always did. He didn't know that U.S. Postal inspectors had set up video surveillance to catch him on tape. As soon as he paid for the shipping and left, the packages were seized. It was enough for the police to get a search warrant.

Now on this wintry morning, Kneller was taking a nap when a half dozen police cars pulled up to his quiet residential complex. The cops holding a search warrant found more than they had bargained for. Kneller collected weapons—his apartment was filled with three Imperial Chinese swords, brass knuckles, a 9mm Glock, a 12-gauge Browning White Lightning shotgun, a pair of Walther sidearms, and a Bersa Thunder semi-automatic pistol. But it was steroids the police had come to find, and they got their warrant's worth. Inside the kitchen, agents found three two-gallon gasoline drums filed with a liquid they would later identify as "suspected steroids." They also discovered 242,060 capsules, 4,578 grams of a white powder, a machine to cap bottles, and labels bearing the name Red Star.

Kneller was dragged off to the local jail.[1] And as he was sitting in his cell, a thought about Dan Duchaine struck him: "How stupid can I be? I'm doing the same things Dan did, all over again. I can't get out from under his shadow. He's probably looking down—or up—at me right now."

COLUMBUS, OHIO
March 5, 2006

After two-and-a-half years in office, Arnold Schwarzenegger was hoping his poll numbers had finally bottomed out. In his first

---

1 In April 2007, Kneller pleaded guilty to 45 counts of steroid possession and distribution and gun possession charges and was sentenced to two years and one day in jail.

few months, he had made good on his promise to be a populist governor. He had tackled California's runaway worker's compensation program and tried to trim its stubborn budget deficits. But in those heady early months, he had also acted like one of his movie characters by picking reckless fights with his state's most powerful unions and its Democratic-led legislature. He sought ballot initiatives to cap education spending, lengthen the time it took teachers to get tenure, and curb the ways unions used dues to back political campaigns. When those initiatives came to a vote the previous November, his policies were so roundly defeated that *Los Angeles Times* political writers Michael Finnegan and Robert Salladay said, "his image as an agent of the popular will" was "shattered."

With his approval rating hovering at 40 percent, Schwarzenegger was glad to take a break from Sacramento and travel to a place where he could truly feel at home—his 18th annual fitness expo in Columbus.

Schwarzenegger had to make a few concessions to his political career. After his multimillion dollar publishing deal with American Media was revealed in the summer of 2005, he signed a bill that banned the use of dietary supplements by California's 700,000 high school athletes. (It expanded on a bill Schwarzenegger had vetoed the year before, banning the sale of Andro to minors.) He also announced he was severing his financial ties to the Arnold Classic.

But Schwarzenegger wasn't about to abandon the expo altogether. On the contrary, he was trying to repackage it, much as he was trying to repackage himself politically. The expo hall was noticeably smaller than in years past (despite an announced count of 650 vendors) and a vast new space was devoted to what he now called The Arnold Sports Festival. Fresh-faced kids were tumbling on gym mats, fencing, dancing on balance beams, and practicing archery, all while their parents looked on approvingly.

While Schwarzenegger tried to maintain this balancing act at the Classic, in Sacramento, the author of the anti-supplement bills he signed, Jackie Speier, was issuing a press release eviscerating him for being in Ohio. "Governor Schwarzenegger, whether or not he likes it, is a role model for our youth," she wrote. "The Arnold Classic glorifies steroids and performance enhancing supplements. Going to this event sends impressionable young people the wrong message. Now, more than ever, teens deserve coaches, role models, and policies that actively discourage teens' use of these substances. The governor is setting a bad example and he should be ashamed of himself."

The previous evening, as he crowned the winner of the Classic, a 36-year-old Floridian named Dexter Jackson, the governor felt a million miles away from Speier's taunts. But it was inevitable that politics would catch up with him. On this day he was hosting a "training seminar" in which anyone who paid $50 could listen to him speak for 45 minutes. Toward the end of the session, the father of a 15-year-old boy asked an unexpected question: His son had been lifting for three years. What supplements did the governor think were okay for the boy to take?

At that moment, the artifice disappeared and Schwarzenegger was open and candid. "I think we have to be very careful to teach our kids not to rely on anything with steroids base or take steroids or any kind of enhancement like that," he began. But in a colloquy that was described as "rambling" by one reporter, he added that there are some "addicts" in the sport who still use them, saying it's probably all right as long as they are adults and "as long as they know there are risks involved."

SCOTTSDALE, ARIZONA

April 19, 2006

While Barry Bonds was closing in on the all-time home run record, Jeff Novitzky was notching a record of his own: most search warrants served by an IRS agent in a sports investigation.

The previous September, he had delivered one to the Illinois lab of Patrick Arnold—finally putting the chemist out of his anticipatory misery. The indictment that resulted was a capstone to the BALCO case. Arnold had created three of the most exotic steroids ever to filter through the underground—Norbolethone, THG, and a little-noticed successor, DMT, also known as Madol—but they had all been rendered obsolete.[2] Now the agent was sitting in his car outside of the red-tile roofed home on East Fanfol Lane, hoping to do the same thing with growth hormone in baseball.

Until this moment, the only cheating that pitcher Jason Grimsley was known for involved an incident at Chicago's Comiskey Park, when his Cleveland Indians teammate, Albert Belle, was caught using a corked bat. After the bat was confiscated, Grimsley had crawled through an air vent connecting the clubhouse to the umpire's dressing room and secretly switched it for one that was uncorked. As Grimsley would later tell writer Buster Olney, "That was one of the biggest adrenaline rushes I've ever experienced."

Grimsley was just as candid when talking about the new addition to Major League Baseball's drug-testing policy—amphetamines. "There are some things that don't need to be in the game," he told reporters at spring training. "But there are things that have been in the game a long time. It's almost like they're trying to change everything about baseball. It's become sterilized."

Still, the players were doing their best to adapt to life without "greenies" and other pick-me-ups. A shift had already begun with some teams, a shift away from clubhouse dealers and shadowy trainers to anti-aging clinics that were already drawing in so many average Americans. Over the winter, former first baseman David Segui had raved to Grimsley about a "wellness clinic" in Florida he had been going to for regular doctor-prescribed injections of human growth hormone because he had been diagnosed as having

---

2 Arnold eventually served three months in prison and three months home confinement for a conspiracy to distribute steroids conviction.

a biologically low supply. "If you're going to do this, you should do it right," Segui said.

It was perfectly reasonable advice, one friend telling another to go to a doctor and not to mess with growth hormone that could be counterfeit or toxic. But Grimsley chose to go elsewhere, and after learning about a shipment that was heading to his home, Novitzky had it intercepted by postal police. Now Novitzky was watching as an undercover postal inspector delivered it to the home on East Fanfol Lane.

The pitcher answered his door, signed for the package, and then disappeared back inside. Novitzky then got out of his car and, flanked by agents from the IRS and FBI, walked up to the house and rang the doorbell again. This time, Grimsley's wife answered and he asked for her husband. When Grimsley appeared, Novitzky showed him the search warrant and gave him a choice: Come with us or we'll search your house. With friends still inside, Grimsley chose the former.

According to an affidavit that was later filed in federal court, Grimsley confessed to many things—about how often he obtained the HGH, about amphetamines, about steroids. But unlike the BALCO case, this wasn't about designer steroids. This was about something that raised questions of everyday health. If a baseball player was going to an anti-aging clinic to keep himself healthy—not to add 30 pounds of muscle—did that actually constitute cheating? What happened if that player requested a legal waiver, known as a therapeutic use exemption? Would it be cheating then?

And what happened if not just a couple, but scores of players started requesting such waivers? Was baseball ready to police such a rapidly changing hormonal playing field?

Was any sport?

COLORADO SPRINGS, COLORADO
July 2006

With the BALCO case starting to recede from the headlines, the people who made their living from the anti-doping fight were being forced to ask themselves what they should do next.

In many ways, BALCO was a gift. It put the war on doping in the public's consciousness, and worries about the tactics used to advance that war on hold. But three years after the discovery of THG, the complaints were starting to come up again. Dick Pound of the World Anti-Doping Agency, for example, was coming under withering criticism for a strange episode involving cyclist Lance Armstrong. French scientists had been conducting tests for the doping drug EPO and had obtained urine samples from the 1999 Tour de France to do it. The one condition of their research was that they keep the identities of the riders anonymous. In a move that violated WADA's rules, Pound demanded coded numbers for the samples—a first step to identifying the riders that had provided them. The second step came when a reporter for the French newspaper *L'Equipe* obtained a master list that matched the numbers to the names. With that list and the secret memo, the reporter was able to determine that Armstrong was one of the riders whose urine had been found to contain synthetic EPO. (Armstrong has consistently denied doping allegations.)

The incident shed an unflattering light on WADA. Above all, it showed Pound to be a meddlesome viceroy who was willing—even eager—to break WADA's rules to catch Armstrong. Once the *L'Equipe* article was published, Pound announced that there was "a very high probability" that Armstrong had used EPO during the 1999 Tour. It confirmed the worst fears of many athletes—that the anti-doping police were willing to go to as extreme lengths as their prey to win.[3]

Terry Madden's experience with cycling at the U.S. Anti-Doping Agency was no less controversial. It involved Tyler Hamilton, the blue-eyed cyclist who had glided to gold at the Athens Olympics in 2004, only to be charged with blood doping in Spain a few weeks later. The test that incriminated Hamilton was originally designed to ensure that pregnant women received safe blood transfusions by checking 12 protein markers in donated blood to verify it was a perfect match for the recipient. In Hamilton's case, a sample he had given in Spain showed two markers that had never been seen in his blood before. The conclusion: he had infused someone else's blood to enrich his own.

Hamilton and his Los Angeles attorney, Howard Jacobs, fought the charge fiercely, publicly attacking USADA's science at every turn. One theory they offered was that his mother had carried a twin who had died in utero early in her pregnancy with Tyler, thereby causing the blood of the "vanishing twin" to mix with Hamilton's own. *The New York Times* gave the story an attentive ear, quoting experts as saying that the vanishing twin theory wasn't so farfetched. It wasn't enough, however, to help Hamilton win.

Madden's deputy, Travis Tygart, expertly shepherded their case through the Court of Arbitration for Sport, and Hamilton received a two-year ban. But even in defeat, the essence of Hamilton's defense still resonated: As the science used to catch athletes became more elaborate, the potential for making small mistakes with huge consequences became greater, too.

Madden understood the danger in relying too heavily on science, which was why he was revising the course he had started charting in 2000. Back then, it was all about drug testing. Now he

---

3 On February 2, 2007, the International Olympic Committee censured Pound for remarks that "could have been regarded as likely to impugn the probity" of Armstrong and were inconsistent with the IOC's goals of "a spirit of friendship, solidarity, and fair play." The commission also recommended that Pound be "remind[ed] ... of the obligation to exercise greater prudence ... when making public pronouncements that may affect the reputation of others." ["IOC rebukes Pound for remarks on Armstrong," *Los Angeles Times*, February 10, 2007.]

was working with four different U.S. Attorney's offices and countless law enforcement departments.

"It can't just be about drug testing anymore," Tygart wrote to Madden in a memo mapping out USADA's future.

The conversations that were underway now only magnified what had begun with the BALCO investigation. They envisioned a permanent police force comprised of USADA, the DEA, and the U.S. Customs and Postal services. As imagined, the new organization would permanently weave USADA—with its web of spies, scientists, and sources—into the federal law enforcement fabric.

The memos that Madden was getting from his staff also included an ambitious plan to create a "passport" program in which athletes could voluntarily give blood or urine samples, thereby creating a biological document that would travel with them. The idea was that by giving USADA such information, innocent athletes would have an easier time explaining deviations that cropped up on their tests.

Madden wasn't sure how much of this radical expansion he could achieve, but he was positive that when it came to policing drugs in sport, the next six years were going to look a lot different than the last six.

LOS ANGELES
July 29, 2006

Five months after Howard Jacobs finished representing Tyler Hamilton, he was thinking of giving up doping cases entirely. He had already done more than just about anyone to challenge Terry Madden and USADA. In fact, he was a bulldog at deconstructing the science that the antidopers used to build their cases. In his defense of Hamilton, Jacobs had examined hundreds of documents and unearthed secret e-mails that, he argued, proved scientists had prematurely rushed the blood-doping test that snared Hamilton.[4] Jacobs believed he had discovered so many flaws in the system that when he lost, he wondered whether it was worth even trying to defend athletes against USADA.

He stopped wondering when his cell phone rang with a call from the manager for Hamilton's successor on the Phonak cycling team, the American rider Floyd Landis.

Landis had been all over the papers during the previous week, thanks to his extraordinary performance in the Tour de France. A Spanish police investigation into a Madrid blood doping operation had implicated two top riders, leading to their suspensions and leaving the field open for Landis. After taking the lead midway through, he had suffered one of the great collapses in cycling history by falling more than 10 minutes back during an 11.4-mile climb up the Alps of southeastern France. But in the next stage, Landis rallied just as historically, rocketing 80 miles across the Alps to a win of nearly six minutes. After Landis cruised onto the Champs Élysées to capture the 2006 Tour, his personal coach told reporters, "You don't even need to enjoy sports [to] understand what he did. It's the sort of thing that motivates people in everyday life."

It certainly impressed Jacobs, a former professional triathlete who closely followed the Tour de France. Two days earlier, cycling officials had cryptically announced that one of the riders had failed a drug test. Now Landis's manager was calling to tell Jacobs, "It's Floyd." The champion's testosterone-to-epitestosterone ratio— which by rule was allowed to be no more than 4:1—was a staggering 11:1. "He needs a lawyer."

Jacobs knew Landis from the Hamilton case. Because Hamilton had pushed Landis for the Phonak team, Landis had volunteered to

---

4 Hamilton lost his case before a three-judge panel of arbitrators by a two-to-one margin. The dissenting judge, Christopher Campbell, wrote this about the blood doping test: "The Lausanne laboratory implementing [it] also failed to estimate the rate of false positives.... If the rate of false positives is not accurately calculated, whether an individual such as Mr. Hamilton is likely to have a false positive is mere speculation, a lot of which has taken place in this case."

be a character witness for him. After Landis had testified, Jacobs thought the cyclist was a true gentleman.

He told Landis's manager that he would be happy to help, but he barely had a chance to get started on the case before another bombshell hit. On this very day, the co-holder of track & field's 100-meter world record, Justin Gatlin, announced that he had failed a drug test, as well.

There were many similarities between Gatlin and Landis. Both were regarded as honest and hardworking professionals in their respective sports. But both also competed under clouds. Landis had inherited the lead role on a team that was still tainted by Hamilton. In Gatlin's case, the cloud came from his scandal-ridden coach, Trevor Graham.

Jacobs worried that having two icons implicated within a day of each other was going to feed the public's cynicism about both. But once his head cleared, he wondered if it might not also present an opportunity. Perhaps the public would begin to question the drug testers, just as he had been doing. Maybe they would come around to believing that mistakes did get made.

The irony was that it would take another of Jacobs's clients—the most notorious one of all—to hammer that crucial point home.

Marion Jones was never charged in the BALCO case. Although Victor Conte publicly named her as a THG and HGH user, he never testified against her.[5] That left the 30-year-old Jones free to compete, which she did at the U.S. Track & Field Championships in Indianapolis in June, winning her 14th national title in the 100 meters.

But roughly three weeks after Jacobs took on the Landis case, he received a similar call from Jones's attorney. The A-sample Jones had provided of her urine in Indianapolis had tested positive for synthetic EPO. She, too, needed Jacobs's help.

---

5 At about the same time Madden wanted Conte to testify, Jones was settling a $25 million defamation suit she had filed against him for statements he made in *ESPN The Magazine* and on ABC's 20/20 regarding her alleged use of performance-enhancing drugs.

In a brief conversation with the track star, Jacobs told her not to get her hopes up about what came next. "The B-sample almost always confirms the A," he explained. Still, on August 30, he took a break from his work for Floyd Landis to make the 40-minute drive from his office in Agoura Hills to the Olympic lab at UCLA. Jacobs knew Don Catlin from prior cases; Catlin had even testified on behalf of a Jacobs client who had sued a supplement company. The men chatted amiably, then they got down to the work of retesting her B-sample.

Catlin performed this test as well as anyone in the world. It was the same one he had used to such great effect at the Salt Lake Olympics. As far as Jacobs was concerned, this was going to be a formality. He watched as the seal on the frozen B-sample was broken and as Catlin's staff started to thaw it. The work was so painstaking that Jacobs excused himself after an hour, leaving the rest of the observation to a specialist he had hired for the job.

Six days later, on September 6, Jacobs was in his office, working on Landis's defense, when his fax machine rang. He looked over to see a cover page from USADA curling out, followed by the lab report in Jones's case. The results were in: The B-sample didn't match.

Jacobs was dumbfounded. It was the first time he could remember such a spectacular failure. There were many possible explanations, besides Jones's innocence, to explain why the results might have turned out that way. One possibility was that the synthetic EPO in Jones's urine had degraded since the A-test was done, making it nearly unrecognizable.

But Terry Madden couldn't have it both ways. A mismatch was a mismatch. And as distasteful as it must have been for him, he had to sit back and watch Jacobs use Marion Jones as a poster girl for the presumption of innocence.

ANSHAN, CHINA
September 7, 2006

As the United States debated how far it wanted to go to police drugs in sport, something strange was happening in China: a full-fledged anti-doping crackdown.

Acting on a tip a few weeks ago, seven anti-doping officers descended on a training camp in the coastal city of Harbin. This was no ordinary facility. It was being used by students of the Liaoning Shenyang Athletics School—an institution known for its most famous teacher: Ma Junren, the father of Ma's Army.

After Ma was removed from the Sydney Olympics for doping offenses in 2000, he had returned to his native Anshan to become deputy chief of the province's Liaoning Provisional Sports Bureau. Ma was now officially retired, but according to the tip received by the authorities, doping was still prevalent in Anshan.

Late in the morning of August 8, the police who descended on the training camp found its staffers openly injecting 10 student-athletes between the ages of 15 and 18. The police then threw open a refrigerator, where they found 25 bottles of EPO, nine bottles of testosterone, and 17 bottles of unknown substances. Finally, they made their way to the headmaster's office, where the real mother lode was stored: 300 more doses of EPO, nine more bottles of testosterone, and 141 bottles of steroids.

Unlike years past, when the whole incident might have been covered up, the central government demanded a full accounting from the Anshan Sports Bureau. The still shell-shocked head of the bureau told the Xinhua General News Service, "We support the decisions and anti-doping stance by the General Administration of Sport and the Chinese Olympic Committee, but we don't understand why the issue was revealed to media before the investigation was concluded."

Nor was the government finished with its surprises.

It was also announcing the results of random tests given during various sports meets in August. Of the more than 250 tests given, 78 athletes had their samples analyzed and four had flunked. It might not have seemed like a shocking number—especially since the quartet competed in weightlifting and wrestling—but for a society that carefully managed its media, it sent an unmistakable message: Chinese authorities had watched what had happened to America during the BALCO affair. And even though their economy was responsible for much of the world's steroid supply, they did not want to be similarly embarrassed when the Olympic Games opened in Beijing in August 2008.

LOS ANGELES
October 1, 2006

"Bar-ry! Bar-ry! Bar-ry!"

Barry Bonds ducked out of the visitors' dugout and waved to the Dodger faithful. In the San Francisco Giants' last game of the year—perhaps his last in a Giants uniform—the 42-year-old superstar ripped a double into right field to lead off the sixth inning, allowing manager Felipe Alou to call for a pinch runner. Once he had returned to the dugout, Bonds heard the 42,831 fans demand a curtain call and he obliged them.

Although his Giants ended the season with a 2-13 record in the final 15 games, Bonds was playing as if he didn't have a care in the world. The previous week in Milwaukee, he hit his 733rd home run, breaking the National League record and putting him 23 long balls away from breaking Hank Aaron's all-time record. No one in baseball knew what to say about that impending milestone, including the Hammer himself. "What am I going to do about it?" Aaron said at an awards ceremony bearing his name. "I have no time to think about it."

It was hard to imagine IRS agent Jeff Novitzky saying the

same thing. All summer long, a debate raged in the San Francisco U.S Attorney's office about whether to ask a grand jury to bring a perjury indictment against Bonds. One group of prosecutors felt they had evidence enough to prove Bonds had lied when he testified that he didn't know his trainer, Greg Anderson, was giving him steroids. The other camp, led by U.S. Attorney Kevin Ryan, felt that more evidence was still needed and they tried to get it by issuing a new subpoena for Anderson (who had just completed his three-month sentence in the BALCO case). But the trainer held fast, refusing to testify. His stand earned him a 15-day sentence for contempt of court.

Ryan's biggest cases to date involved violent street gangs, so he wasn't going to allow himself to be pushed around by one gym rat. After the term of the sitting grand jury expired, a new grand jury was empanelled with an 18-month term. On August 17, Anderson once again refused to testify. And once again, a judge ordered him back to jail—though this time with a term that had the potential to last until January 2008.

With Anderson sitting silently behind bars, Barry Bonds was free to consider a future that his agent insisted was still bright. "I believe all 30 teams would be interested in him, based on the revenue he could bring to [a] franchise," his agent, Jeff Borris, told reporters about the 2007 season.

In the meantime, Ryan's prosecutors tied up a few other loose ends. The first involved Trevor Graham, the track coach who had blown the whistle on THG. In November 2006, he had been indicted for lying to investigators about his relationship with a man who peddled performance-enhancing drugs. In December, cyclist Tammy Thomas would also be indicted on charges of lying to a federal grand jury when she claimed that she had never received steroids from BALCO chemist Patrick Arnold. (Both have pleaded not guilty to charges of perjury and misleading investigators.)

But despite all the testimony, all the man-hours spent digging into the dark corners of sport, no professional athlete had ever been charged with committing a crime.

GUADALAJARA, MEXICO

November 22, 2006

On the first anniversary of Alberto Saltiel-Cohen's arrest, John Romano got on yet another flight from his home in Florida to Guadalajara. The first time was in January, when he had been to Tijuana to determine the effect that Operation Gear Grinder had had on the steroid trade.

In January, Romano had found that its *farmacias* were full of fakes. Real high-dose veterinary "gear" was so scarce that it cost as much as legitimate European pharmaceutical steroids. That was something Romano had never seen before. The DEA was to be congratulated. But a few weeks earlier, an old friend named Hector called him to say, "The hole has been filled." According to the former Mr. Mexico, the *cho-cho* was flowing freely again. Romano boarded a flight to Mexico to see for himself.

When he landed in Guadalajara, Romano was picked up by his publishing business partner, the owner of a local Gold's Gym, and brought to their publishing office where Hector and another dealer, Guzman, were waiting.

"There are some really good vet drugs coming over from Spain and Italy," Hector began. "Tons of it—Sustanon, trenbolone, Equipoise, Primobolan, oxandrolone, Winstrol. As much as you want." He opened a box to show Romano labels from all over the world: India, Thailand, Turkey, Italy, Bulgaria, Argentina, Hungary, Austria, Spain, and even Mexico.

"In my gym alone, the trainers move $60,000 a month," their host said.

Romano turned to Guzman to ask where his stuff was coming from. "If you can get it at the *farmacia,* you can get it from me," he told Romano. "But with no prescription. I can get anything else, too, besides the *cho-cho.* Viagra, Valium, diet pills, Prozac, anything you want. Even crazy shit, like OxyContin."

Romano wanted to know if any of it made it to the United States, but Guzman waved off the thought. "Hell no. That would be crazy. I make plenty of money here and have no risk."

So where were the steroids entering America coming from?

Hector leaned in and dropped his voice. "There are smaller labs popping up that make stuff for the border," he said. "I know of one lab in Nuevo Laredo that sends everything to the States. There are other labs starting up around Mexico City making drugs for the States, too."

Romano thought about how far Mexico had come since Dan Duchaine began smuggling two decades ago. It was finally what The Guru had envisioned, a gateway for steroids from all around the world to reach America. On the way home, Romano began writing the piece that would appear in the February 2007 issue of *Muscular Development:*

> *The question that begs to be asked is whether the fifth-ranked entrepreneurial country in the world is going to wave off a $56-million-a-year market. Of course not. What happened was a shift in the process, so the money could still be made. In fact, it seems as if Operation Gear Grinder was the catalyst for the underground Mexican economy to revamp itself. In so doing, it appears they have made some improvements. I'll bet when the DEA runs those numbers again when it plans its next battle, they'll find the market has significantly grown.*

20

GROWING PAINS

February 16, 2007 - June 27, 2007

SYDNEY, AUSTRALIA

February 16-19, 2007

Just as Linda Hamilton had redefined body image for women in *Terminator 2*, Sylvester Stallone was trying to do the same thing for 60-year-old men with *Rocky Balboa*, the sixth film in his signature franchise. The storyline wasn't going to win any screenwriting awards: Rocky decides to step into the ring after seeing a computer simulation of himself fighting the current champion on ESPN. But that didn't matter. Fans didn't go to Rocky movies for the plot. They went for the same reason they would visit Rome: to see how the ruins were holding up. And, by all accounts, Sly was doing just fine. Writing in *The New York Times*, Stephen Holden observed: "Mr. Stallone's body is a sight. A weightlifter's slab of aged meat, knotted with tiny hard veins popping out of the shoulders, it is just this side of muscle-bound and somewhat grotesque. It is something you might see hung in the window of a steak house and wonder what kind of carnivore would order such a leathery, sinewy carcass."

Since its release in late December, *Rocky Balboa* was doing respectable business for MGM. On an international tour that included a red carpet walk in London's Leicester Square, Stallone was receiving enthusiastic receptions. Up ahead was a premiere in Sydney. As he stepped off a Qantas flight, he handed a Customs agent an incoming visitor card that asked whether he was bringing in any "medicines, steroids, firearms, weapons, or any kind of illicit drugs." Stallone circled the word "no."

Unfortunately for him, an alert airport employee discovered that his answer wasn't entirely true. When Stallone's luggage was randomly X-rayed, the machine turned up 48 vials of human growth hormone.

The discovery led Customs officials to escort Stallone to a detention area, where the actor tried to explain why he had filled out the visitor card as he did. After Sydney, he explained, he was heading to Myanmar (formerly Burma) to film his fourth Rambo movie. "Doing Rambo is hard work and I'm going to be in Burma for a while," he told one Customs officer. "Where do you think I am going to get this stuff in Burma?"

Two hours later, Stallone was released and given permission to attend the Australian premiere of his movie at an open-air screen overlooking Sydney Harbor on Saturday. But, he was told, he should expect a visit by Australian Customs officials with a notice for him to appear in court. When reporters got wind of his detention on Sunday, Stallone tried to keep the whole affair low-key. "I do know [why I was stopped] but I can't tell you," he told Sydney's *Daily Telegraph*. "To [Customs] it's major, but it's really minor stuff. I just made a mistake ... I misunderstood a few things and we are going through the process."

Apparently, Stallone wasn't done misunderstanding the Australian drug laws. When Customs agents arrived at the swank Park Hyatt the next day to deliver the court notice, they noticed something strange by Stallone's hotel window: There was Rocky himself (some reports claim it was members of his entourage), feverishly throwing pills out of the hotel. While one group of agents rushed up to his room, and another was dispatched to search a private jet that Stallone had waiting for him at the airport, a third went to recover the discarded pills. They were later analyzed and found to be testosterone cypionate.

As it happens, Stallone was getting some very good medical advice. A study by Sydney's own Garvan Institute found that HGH taken alone doesn't do much except increase fluid retention. However, when taken in conjunction with testosterone, the study found that HGH had a demonstrable effect in one category: sprinting power. Of course, the authors of the study noted that any athlete using them in tandem stood a greater chance of getting caught since drug tests routinely pick up testosterone.

But actors didn't get tested for drugs, did they?

The question of who advised Stallone was answered when the case eventually came to trial. (He would eventually plead guilty to two counts of importing and possessing prohibited substances.) Although Stallone couldn't produce any prescriptions for the drugs he was carrying, he did submit a note from his doctor, who attested to the fact that he was taking them under medical supervision. The doctor's name was familiar to anyone who had hung around Lyle Alzado at the end of his life—it was Alzado's personal physician, Robert Huizenga.

ORLANDO, FLORIDA
February 27, 2007

Eugene Bolton, a former semi-pro football player, slid the envelope across the table to his lunch mate, a beautiful obstetrician with a side practice in anti-aging medicine. Inside the envelope was $1,750—payment for easy work. According to Bolton, all the doctor had done was sign prescription orders for people she had never met and could scarcely even call patients. The meeting had been arranged by a third person at the table, the business manager for Signature, a pharmacy down the street.

Signature belonged to a little-known, but lucrative corner of the pharmaceutical industry called compounding pharmacies. Instead of selling name-brand drugs, compounding pharmacies bought bulk raw materials from around the world and then mixed their own generic drugs. There are hundreds of compounding pharmacies in the United States, but Signature had a special niche. As Bolton knew all too well, it supplied a national network of "wellness centers" that weren't nearly as wholesome as they sounded. The 6-foot-7, 345-pound Bolton called his suburban Houston outfit Cellular Nucleonic Advantage, but the name was just window dressing. He advertised in custom car magazines for people who wanted to get cheap and easy prescriptions, then took orders with his girlfriend over the phone.

Once a customer was on board, Bolton sent his or her prescription request to a friendly doctor who would sign it, often for as little as $25. The last stop on the drug chain was Signature, which would fill the prescription and send it back to the customer.

According to a report prepared for the World Anti-Doping Agency, an estimated $2 billion worth of HGH has been sold worldwide, and places like Signature were a big reason why.

The company imported the raw powder from China through a local businessman. (His main job was, of all things, building stone fountains for mansions, but he went to China frequently enough to have made other connections.) And it was all legal, or at least mostly legal. Unlike steroids, growth hormone wasn't on the federal register of controlled substances; the only way an individual could get in trouble was by not having a prescription.

According to the information Bolton provided to authorities, that's where he came in, and why Signature's business manager was eager to help him. In an effort to help him clear more prescriptions,

Bolton claimed the executive suggested he strike up a relationship with Claire Godfrey, the anti-aging doctor who also worked as a medical correspondent for Fox TV. The money he was handing over was for 30 prescription forms that she had signed.[1]

What Bolton's lunch mates didn't know was that the ex-lineman was wired for sound. Laws about doctor-patient relationships vary from state to state, but New York has one of the toughest: doctors must see a patient before writing a prescription. Agents working for the District Attorney in Albany, New York, had been looking into doctors who were writing e-mail prescriptions without face-to-face meetings when they stumbled on Bolton's operation. Cornering him, they said that he could cooperate in a case against Signature or take his chances going to jail. Bolton cooperated and the transcript of this lunch proved to be exactly what the lawmen needed.

On February 27, they would descend on Signature and arrest Bolton's two lunch mates, along with Signature's owners, a married pair of Orlando pharmacists who had done $36 million worth of business in 2006. (While the principals in the Signature case would plead not guilty, Bolton and his girlfriend both accepted felony charges of filing false prescriptions.)

During the raid, the agents would also cart away box loads of patient records that showed Sylvester Stallone was hardly alone in using HGH. One invoice showed that Signature shipped growth hormone to a New York hotel room that was occupied by a member of a major pop star's touring band. Another reportedly showed that Gary Matthews, a 32-year-old outfielder for the Los Angeles Angels, ordered some as well, from a pharmacy in Alabama. (In a statement issued two weeks after the first report, Matthews insisted, "I have never taken HGH.")

The NFL would also discover that a doctor for the Pittsburgh Steelers purchased $150,000 in performance enhancers with his

---

1 Dr. Godfrey eventually pleaded guilty to criminal diversion of prescription medications and was sentenced to five years' probation.

credit card. (Though dropped from the team's roster, the doctor has not been accused of any wrongdoing and has stated that the HGH he ordered is intended for his older patients.)

Beyond that, Arnold Schwarzenegger would be left red-faced on the weekend of the 2007 Arnold Expo when reporters informed him that the man he had just crowned winner of his Arnold Classic, Victor Martinez, had bought steroids from a clinic involved in the case.[2] The governor's spokesman was left to reply, "Clearly, steroid use is something he is very strongly opposed to."[3]

SHANGHAI, CHINA

Spring 2007

Nothing in the pharmaceutical executive's appearance suggested that he was one of China's largest producers of HGH— nothing, that is, except the pained expression that crossed his face when he was asked about the arrest of Sylvester Stallone.

Business had been good lately. His company was among China's fast growing biotech firms and the rows of cubicles outside his office attested to the growing size of his sales staff. Indeed, the executive saw what he was doing as a kind of public service for the people of China.

Other drug companies made growth hormone, but the price was astronomical—in some cases as much as $80 a unit. And it didn't have to be. In 2005, Swiss-based Serono labs and its U.S. subsidiaries paid the third largest healthcare fraud recovery in American history—$704 million—after evidence emerged that it was profiting off a drug approved by the FDA solely to treat AIDS wasting syndrome. Once the demand for the drug abated

---

2 Martinez has not been charged and is not named in the indictments. He claimed he was buying testosterone because he had been diagnosed as having low levels by a clinic involved in the larger investigation that had prescribed it. The clinic owners have pleaded not guilty to submitting prescriptions for steroids without a medical need.

3 The headlines didn't end there. Eleven wrestlers, including several WWE superstars, were caught in a parallel investigation of a Mobile, Alabama, company called Applied Pharmacy.

because of the advent of protease inhibitors, Serono created a fraudulent system for measuring body cell mass that qualified thousands of otherwise unqualified patients. This in turn led to Medicaid reimbursements for six-week treatments costing as much as $21,000 each. In the end, scores of patients wound up selling the HGH that they didn't need to bodybuilders and other athletes, simultaneously padding Serono's profits and fueling the black market.

The Chinese executive portrayed himself as a pharmaceutical patriot, making HGH for as low as a dollar a unit for his country's needy: children with dwarfism, burn victims, people with AIDS. "The American price is too high for the Chinese people," he explained. "We give them hope."

But Stallone's arrest for possession of HGH had brought unwanted attention to his industry. Now the FDA had put certain brands of Chinese HGH on a special watch list so that any shipments directly to the United States could be seized and destroyed.

The executive said he hoped to be seen as reputable by the American government, not as a rogue, which was why he recently stopped selling directly to the U.S. through his Web site. "I want the FDA to know we want to be legal," he said. But then he added that he couldn't control where his products went once they were sold to the hospital supply wholesalers who distributed it around China. "The demand is very great," he allowed.

What concerned him most was the explosion of counterfeit growth hormone, much of it sold under legitimate brand names, including his own. The technology to manufacture HGH is difficult, but once mastered, it can be easily reproduced. "Some of the people making this have worked for me before," he said knowingly. "But what can I do? They could be in India, Pakistan, maybe even Moscow. They can be anywhere."

To the police in Hanover, New Jersey, it was about to become clear that China's performance enhancement pipeline didn't stop with wellness clinics and anti-aging doctors. It was also fueling a new breed of underground steroid labs that supplied Main Street America.

That was evident when they decided to pay a visit to Anthony Cuppari, a volunteer assistant coach for the Hornets of Hanover Park High School.

In the fall of 2006, New Jersey became the first state to mandate steroid monitoring, ordering that playoff teams be randomly tested at the start of the new academic year. But the prospect of testing hadn't stopped whispers from circulating about the Hornets. After the team crushed its opening day opponent 42-0, the team's coach, Dan Gregory, told the Morristown *Daily Record*, "The numbers in the weight room are better than any ever."

Looking at game film before a fall 2006 match-up with the Hornets, the coaches at rival Chatham High could see that was no idle boast. These kids were huge. And so was Cuppari, an ex-Hornets running back who worked as personal trainer at a gym in Florham Park. Because of his size, he was impossible to miss prowling the sideline.

The Chatham coaches couldn't help but be suspicious. But those suspicions might have remained idle if not for one thing: Just before New Jersey was enacting its steroid testing program, Morris County police arrested 54 people in a probe of prescription painkillers sales around Hanover Park High and two other area high schools. During the course of that probe, they learned that steroids were being peddled along with the painkillers.

After a two-month undercover operation, the police obtained search warrants for the home of Cuppari and a friend named

Michael Dente. In the first house, they found steroids, GHB, cocaine, and what was later described as "items necessary to the manufacturing process." In the second, they found a fully functional drug lab, complete with a pill press and raw materials from China and elsewhere used to make steroids, Cialis, Viagra, and GHB. Both men were charged with second-degree felony counts involving conspiracy to manufacture the drugs and several counts of drug distribution. (The cases are still pending.)

As the sweep broadened, 16 people were arrested, including a 17-year-old Hornets player who allegedly bought GHB—which can be used to mask steroids. A 35-year-old bodybuilder allegedly loaned his drug-making expertise to the crew.

And just like that, Hanover, New Jersey, was forced to answer the same question that had already been asked in Colleyville, Texas—the same question that was destined to confront more and more communities: Was it time to make steroid testing in schools even stronger?

In Orlando, Florida, a police officer working on the Signature case left little doubt that something had to be done. "We're finding a lot of kids, 15, 16 [ordering steroids]," he told the *Palm Beach Post*. "It's a simple thing. They get a prepaid credit card at Albertson's, and suddenly they're playing better basketball and their parents don't know why."

Meanwhile, a Florida legislator had proposed a pilot program to test one percent of the state's 59,000 football, basketball, and weightlifting athletes. Around the same time, the lieutenant governor of Texas was pushing a bill to target 22,000 of his state's 733,000 public school students.

In the midst of all this, researchers at the University of Minnesota released a little-noticed report that raised a question about whether all the legislating was heading in the right direction.

Researchers there surveyed 2,516 middle and high school students in 1999, and then followed up again in 2004. What they discovered was that those who were in high school in 1999 were three times less likely to use steroids when they became young adults. In other words, they experimented for a time, got tired of the novelty, and moved on. The survey also noted that most of the use was casual. Among the 1,130 boys who were tracked, only two—or .17 percent—reported using them every day. Slightly more than half of those who used said they did so "a few times in the past year."

What was particularly striking about the survey was that all those who admitted experimenting with steroids weren't using them exclusively for sports. Both boys *and girls* reported trying steroids because they wanted better bodies, albeit for opposite reasons: The boys felt they were too thin, while the girls felt overweight.

Given that, did it really make sense for school districts to get into contentious and costly biological wars with their students? The lead author of the study, Patricia van den Berg, considered the question: "It depends on society's aim," she said. "If the aim is its making sports clean, then the answer may be yes. But if the aim is to affect adolescent health, it may be wiser to put the same money into seat belt education, since automobile accidents are a leading cause of death among teenagers."

In the end, it all seemed to come down to what Lori Lewis had discovered in Colleyville: The best line of defense is parents who want to know the truth, and coaches who are willing to stand up for it.

LOS ANGELES
March 2007

After a quarter century as America's leading steroid hunter, Don Catlin understood the limits of testing better than anyone. When he began his anti-doping career, he tried to be equal parts detective and doctor, which was why he often skated around Venice Beach to eavesdrop on the bodybuilders. He also tried to get his clients to think unconventionally. In the late 1980s, for instance, he floated a novel idea with the NFL. They drug-tested their athletes more than any other sport. So why not keep that data over time, creating a biological scrapbook for each athlete? That way, if the athlete had an anomalous reading, it could be flagged, examined, and deciphered. Instead of waiting for drug tests to catch the cheaters, the NFL could use records it *already had* to see preemptively if something was amiss.

A simple enough idea, but it went nowhere.

An American cycling team called Slipstream/Chipotle had recently implemented a variation of the plan. But as far as Catlin was concerned, it came two decades too late. And at 68, he didn't have another two decades to spend waiting for results.

Thanks to a joint project undertaken by the U.S. Anti-Doping Agency and the NFL, a new drug-testing lab had just opened in Salt Lake City, and Catlin was more than willing to leave the daily grind of drug testing to the newcomers. He was more energized about a new research center he had opened a mile or so away from the UCLA campus. It already had $500,000 in financing from Major League Baseball to determine whether a urine test for HGH was feasible. (Catlin didn't think so, but he was willing to give it a shot.)

And so Catlin sat down in his office to type an e-mail to USADA's Terry Madden. It was a perfect time to say, "It's been an honor to serve you, but I am resigning my position as the director of the UCLA Olympic Analytical Lab." After he pressed the send key, he gathered his lab's 50 employees in his office for an impromptu goodbye speech.

"When I started this lab, drug testing was just a means to an end," he told his staff. "Now I'm hoping to find a new means to that end. Because the old way—chasing, collecting, and analyzing—just isn't working. No matter how hard we work, there are just too many ways around it."

COLORADO SPRINGS, COLORADO

March 2007

When Terry Madden received Don Catlin's resignation letter, he understood the need to move on. A week earlier, he had announced that he, too, was stepping down. With the second of his three children heading to college, and a third entering eighth grade, Madden was ready to leave USADA in the hands of the people who had helped build it.

But first, there was one more case to win—the case involving Tour de France champion Floyd Landis. Unlike most other accused dopers who disappeared from public view after they were charged, Landis seemed to be everywhere. With the help of seasoned public relations advisors, he was blitzing the media and barnstorming through fundraising benefits. The presidential primary season may have been heating up, but Landis was running the best campaign in the nation.

And it was working. In February 2007, MSNBC polled more than 35,000 people and found that 68 percent of them thought Landis was "totally innocent of doping." Plenty of athletes had attacked USADA before. Marion Jones had once famously called it a "kangaroo court." But Landis was actually getting the public to listen. His boldness was evident in a February interview that he'd given to Elliott Almond of the San Jose *Mercury News.* "The big problem with anti-doping agencies [is that] they have no financial incentive to get to the truth," he said. "They have an incentive to get the riders.... If they catch someone in my position they take that and go to the government and ask for more money. The problem is at the root in the whole system."

Landis had reframed the case. Rather than defend individual guilt, he was challenging the legitimacy of the system that Madden had painstakingly helped to build. Madden would retire in seven months, but his successors, led by the smart and ambitious Travis

Tygart, would have to show that the agency could withstand a little sunlight as it continued to probe deeper into the shadows.

MALIBU, CALIFORNIA
May 17, 2007

Howard Jacobs had a spring in his step as he arrived at Pepperdine Law School for the fourth day of testimony in Floyd Landis's arbitration trial. Things had been going well enough for Jacobs to be cautiously optimistic about his decision to convince Landis to open his hearing to the public. Yesterday, he had placed a copy of the World Anti-Doping Agency's rules before the arbitrators and pointed out one particular provision: the one that stated that officials of any WADA-accredited lab could not testify in court against the work of any other lab. Then he watched the eyes of one of the arbitrators, Chris Campbell, grow wide. "You've got a code of ethics of laboratory directors that essentially states that they can't point out the mistakes of the lab?" he said with evident surprise.

Jacobs wanted the arbitrators—as well as the public—to be shocked; his whole defense centered on discrediting the Paris lab that had accused Landis of doping. The attorney believed that the lab's director ran a shockingly loose operation, trusting the most sensitive machines to young women with little or no experience. Two of them had already testified, and Jacobs felt his cross-examinations had shown that they were ill prepared for the complex work of measuring testosterone levels with a gas chromatograph combustion isotope ratio mass spectrometer.[4]

Jacobs felt that if he could just establish reasonable doubt on the science, he was sure his client could finish off the job by testifying to his own character. After all, Landis had a good story to sell about

---

4 The essence of his case involved one of four things measured by the lab—a metabolite of testosterone known as 5A. The lab concluded that a low level was proof of doping. But an expert whom Jacobs consulted testified that the reading was skewed: no study had ever found that 5A varied by more than two parts per million from its metabolic cousin, 5B; in Landis's case, the variance was four.

growing up as a Mennonite in Lancaster County, Pennsylvania. As a retired doctor from Lancaster told ESPN.com, "I've treated thousands of Mennonite people. And I don't know I've ever caught one in a lie. That man [Landis] is innocent."

But something Jacobs had heard on his way to court was bothering him. Something about a prank that Landis's manager, Will Geoghegan, had played the night before on Greg LeMond, the three-time Tour de France champion. LeMond was scheduled to testify about a conversation he had had with Landis shortly after Landis's A-sample drug test results were reported in the press. The men barely knew one another, but during a tense conversation, LeMond told Landis that if he was truly guilty, he should "help himself" and the sport by coming clean.

According to LeMond, Landis said, "What good would it do? If I did, it would destroy a lot of my friends and hurt a lot of people."

Before they hung up, LeMond added a strikingly personal postscript: He confided that he had been sexually abused as a child, and said he hoped that Landis wasn't going to be as haunted as he was about the secret he was keeping.

When Jacobs approached Geoghegan to ask what exactly had happened with LeMond the night before, the manager tried laughing it off. But Jacobs was aghast when Geoghegan conceded that after drinking a few beers, he had called LeMond, pretending to be his uncle and raising the issue of the sexual abuse. It was all just a silly joke, Geoghegan explained. Jacobs felt less than assured.

When LeMond began his testimony, it was instantly clear to Jacobs and his co-counsel, Maurice Suh, how bad things really were. LeMond began by testifying to the original conversation. Then he was asked by a USADA prosecutor, "Did you receive a telephone call last night on your cell phone that you understand was connected to your testimony in this case, Mr. LeMond?"

LeMond said that he had, that the caller had told him, "Hi Greg, this is your uncle." And when LeMond asked, "Who is this?" he was told, "I'll be there tomorrow and we can talk about how we used to hide your weenie."

"I got the picture right away," LeMond testified. "I figured this was an intimidation to keep me from coming here."

Jacobs went pale. For three days, reporters had been complaining that the trial was a yawner, with too much obscure science. Now, just as he had been gaining ground for Landis, his manager had given the press exactly the wrong thing to write about.

As Jacobs got up to start his cross-examination, he tried to portray LeMond as a has-been who had previously tried to discredit Lance Armstrong with a similar story of doping. But LeMond's attorney cut him off, saying Armstrong had nothing to do with the case. By the end of the day, the spring in Jacobs's step had disappeared. No one was talking about the French lab he hoped to put on trial. Nor would they.

In the weeks to come, Landis's reputation was hammered further. In a book called *From Lance to Landis*, David Walsh, chief sportswriter of *The Sunday Times* (of London), repeated allegations that Armstrong used performance-enhancing drugs. He also cited an ugly incident that occurred between Armstrong and his former teammate. In 2004, just after Landis announced he was leaving the U.S. Postal team to ride for a rival, Armstrong reportedly took bags of blood that Landis was saving to transfuse himself on rest days and dumped them down the toilet. The alleged episode was described by former teammate Jonathan Vaughters, who claimed he heard it from Landis.[5]

In the face of all this, Armstrong and Landis defended their innocence and each other. At a speaking engagement in Aspen, Armstrong flatly said of Landis, "I don't think he did it." At a separate

---

5   After the release of *From Lance to Landis*, Armstrong issued a statement attacking the veracity of Walsh's book and his previous book on which it was based, saying, "Walsh and his sources are liars." He further stated: "... the *Sunday Times* [of London] published some of Walsh's allegations as excerpts from his previous book *[L.A. Confidential: The Secrets of Lance Armstrong]* and after a series of victories in the British courts, I received a formal apology from the *Sunday Times* for ever re-publishing Walsh's allegations."

appearance, the retired champion went even further, wondering if it was possible to win without being dogged by doping rumors: "What happens if a guy who's considered clean comes along and races as fast as anybody ever has? Well, then he's got to be dirty, too."

An avalanche of new doping disclosures made it hard to feel that any cyclist was getting a raw deal. In May, Denmark's Bjarne Riis, the 1996 Tour winner, admitted that he had used illegal drugs in his quest and was promptly stripped of his yellow jersey. Italian authorities announced that Ivan Basso, runner-up in the 2005 Tour, was cooperating in an ongoing probe of a Madrid doctor after admitting that his blood was in plastic bags that had been seized there. And German investigators continued their probe of nine riders who had been banned from the 2006 Tour, including Jan "The Diesel" Ullrich, after his DNA matched yet more blood seized from the Spanish doctor's clinic. (Ullrich has now retired from racing.)

One could only wonder if the pressure that led to these revelations might one day be duplicated in baseball, a sport that seemed to be in the same state of denial that cycling had been in just a few years earlier.

> CHICAGO
> *May 17, 2007*

Jason Giambi had no idea what kind of trouble he was about to make for himself. He was waiting for a game against the Chicago White Sox to start when Bob Nightengale, a veteran reporter from *USA Today*, asked him about Barry Bonds and steroids. The likeable Yankee designated hitter turned reflective, bringing up a vague apology that he had made two years earlier. "In hindsight, it helped me," he began. "I was wrong for doing that stuff. I know that. But [apologizing] is the best thing that happened. I got it out of the way so that people stopped asking me about it.... With everything else that has gone on, you hardly ever hear my name mentioned now."

Giambi's off-the-cuff remark guaranteed that the exact opposite would happen. George Mitchell, the former senator from Maine, was in the midst of conducting an investigation into baseball about its steroid problem. But after $30 million and 15 months, no athlete, let alone an active player, had come forward openly to discuss it. Giambi brought that wall of silence down on himself when he continued: "What we should have done a long time ago was stand up—players, ownership, everybody—and said, 'We made a mistake.'"

After a frenzied bit of backpedaling, Giambi (and his attorneys) worked out a deal in which he agreed to talk about himself and no one else. But his remarks still hit baseball like a thunderbolt. Honesty about steroids? Greg Anderson was sitting mute in a jail cell, serving his seventh month on contempt charges rather than testify about Barry Bonds. Meanwhile, countless players were biding their time, hoping that they would never have to talk about what they did when everyone else was doing it.

News of Giambi's testimony was coming weeks after another damning incident for baseball—the search warrant that had been served on a former batboy and clubhouse attendant for the New York Mets named Kirk Radomski. The search warrant affidavit alleged that after working for the team from 1985 to 1995, Radomski became an experienced drug courier and expanded his operations after BALCO closed in 2003. An affidavit authored by BALCO investigator Jeff Novitzky claimed that his bank account had "numerous significant deposits from current and former MLB players, as well as some individuals associated with MLB players." As with another infamous affidavit Novitzky wrote—the one having to do with the journeyman pitcher Jason Grimsley—player names were blacked out. (The omissions prompted two lawsuits to disclose them by Hearst and the Associated Press. A Phoenix judge eventually ruled against AP in the Grimsley matter, citing the need to protect an ongoing investigation.)

Ultimately, Radomski pleaded guilty to charges of distribution of controlled substances and money laundering, and was required to cooperate with the Mitchell Commission. He also testified before the same grand jury that was investigating Bonds, guaranteeing that the guessing game of "Who Used?" would stay front-and-center for some time.

Meanwhile, Bonds himself inched ever closer to Hank Aaron's record of 755 home runs. If one thing about his slow march was striking, it was the sheer joylessness of it all. Aaron made clear that he wouldn't attend the record-breaking, while Bud Selig practiced a tortured kind of diplomacy, deflecting questions about whether he would be present when Bonds broke the record.

The morality of the moment mirrored the larger debate over steroids: Was Bonds less of an athlete if he took them? Or was he simply like millions of other Americans who were trying to turn back the clock? Was he cheating? Or was he doing what players had done since the dawn of the game—trying to get an edge?

The questions might have generated a more sympathetic response if Bonds looked like he was having more fun, or at least like he was letting fans have fun with him. But the sullen way he approached Aaron's record made it about him, not about those watching him.

As a result, the 42-year-old slugger mirrored no one in the steroid debate except himself.

NEW YORK CITY

June 27, 2007

The news vendors outside Grand Central hawked the morning editions of *A.M. New York* by shouting its headline: "Roid Rage!" The story referred to Chris Benoit, a member of Vince McMahon's World Wrestling Entertainment troupe who had committed a gruesome crime, killing his wife and seven-year-old son.

Benoit wasn't the most muscular man in the WWE. His claim to fame was his acrobatic leaps off the ring posts and his technical mastery of holds. As such, he appeared to be one of the lucky members of McMahon's traveling circus. Over the past 20 years, at least eight-dozen wrestlers had ended up dead before they turned 50. No one could say for certain that steroids alone were to blame in any of these deaths. Many wrestlers had other addictions—painkillers to keep them going, booze, hard drugs. But steroids put extra stress on a user's heart, forcing it to work harder to pump blood to unnaturally enlarged physiques. And only someone in deep denial would discount a link.

Up until this shocking news, Benoit was seen as a quiet, even sensitive, man, who had been deeply affected by the deaths of his colleagues. But he was hit hardest by the death of his best friend in the business, 38-year-old Eddie Guerrero. The two had been through everything that wrestling could throw at them, and just when they seemed to have it all, Guerrero had died alone in a Minneapolis hotel room from heart failure. Benoit never recovered from the November 2005 loss. At one point, his wife, Nancy, even bought him a diary so he could write "Dear Eddie" letters to the deceased Guerrero.

Benoit's private torments stayed hidden until June 24, when co-workers who were expecting him at an event in Beaumont, Texas, began getting cryptic e-mails alerting them to his "physical location." Concerned about the wrestling star, aides to McMahon called police in Fayetteville, Georgia, asking them to visit Benoit's gated mansion.

The police found a scene of sickening suburban carnage: Nancy had been strangled in their home office with a Bible at her side, while their son, Daniel, lay lifeless on his upstairs bed, still dressed in pajamas amid the posters of his father that adorned the walls of his room and a Bible beside him. Benoit himself was found bare-chested and bloated in his basement gym, having hanged himself from a cable attached to 240 pounds of weights. Inevitably, steroids were found in the house.

As the local district attorney, Scott Ballard, speculated that 'roid rage was "one of the things that we'll be looking at," TV networks filled in the blanks. "Depression, paranoia, and violent outbursts known as 'roid rage are linked with steroid use," an NBC reporter said during the lead-in to a *Today* show segment with McMahon, who was lamely left to beg for patience. "It's all speculation until the toxicology reports come back," he told a visibly skeptical Meredith Vieira.

In the days to come, the story would take several turns that seemed to suggest that the impetus for the crime was obvious. The DEA admitted it had been monitoring Benoit's doctor, who had given him 10-month supplies of steroids every few weeks between May 2006 and May 2007.[6] Benoit's name also turned up on the client lists of Signature, the Orlando compounding pharmacy at the center of the bogus prescription case. The link dramatically expanded the depth of the multistate investigation that had mostly been about aging athletes getting career-extending drugs through the Internet, and included fellow wrestler Kurt Angle (who did not respond to being named), former heavyweight champion Evander Holyfield (who denied using performance-enhancing drugs), and baseball outfielder Gary Matthews.

When the toxicology reports eventually came back, it was determined that Benoit had a heightened level of testosterone in his system (more than 10 times the natural amount), as well as the anti-anxiety drug Xanax and the painkiller hydrocodone. The coroner added, however, that there was nothing to show that steroids had played a part in the deaths.

Fairly or not, Benoit had become a symbol of a Steroid Nation that was out of control. Now steroids were not simply drugs taken

---

6 A DEA spokesman defended its strategy, saying that the agency was quietly building a case against the doctor, Phil Astin, and usually did not prosecute users anyway. After the Benoit incident, Dr. Astin was charged with illegal distribution of prescription drugs. He pleaded not guilty.

by cheaters in professional sports, they were drugs that turned people into raving murderers. Even the word "steroid" itself became an all-purpose, fear-generating rubric—like "terrorism" or "global warming."

It was a grim, fatalistic version of the Steroid Nation that Dan Duchaine had envisioned more than a quarter century earlier when he walked into Gold's Gym for the first time. In those days, Duchaine saw himself as a latter-day Dr. Jekyll, a futurist and a humanist who believed he could unlock human potential through chemistry. In that sense, he was walking the same path as Sigmund Freud, who had proselytized about the benefits of cocaine, and Timothy Leary, who, in the 1960s, urged people to "turn on, tune in, drop out" by taking LSD. And, like his spiritual predecessors, Duchaine believed that he could succeed where the literary Dr. Jekyll had failed. Dan Duchaine believed he could control his elixirs and the Mr. Hydes they unleashed.

He was wrong.

By injecting one tiny corner of California with steroids, Duchaine and his disciples had spread the gospel of performance-enhancing drugs to an entire country. From Gold's in Venice Beach to the BALCO lab in San Francisco, from a high school in Colleyville, Texas, to teenagers in Hanover, New Jersey. Albany. Orlando. Charlotte. Columbus. Today, steroids are everywhere in America.

And Steroid Nation is rapidly becoming part of a larger Steroid World: Mexico, India, Greece, Thailand, Spain, China. Dr. Jekyll can prescribe in any language.

In 1981, Dan Duchaine had a simple idea for a book that would galvanize the new world he wanted to create. The words he helped write in the *Underground Steroid Handbook* sound as urgent today as they did then:

"Although we'll antagonize many of you, we thought we should tell the truth about steroids."

ACKNOWLEDGMENTS

The research for this book began in the fall of 2005 with a wine-tasting tour through the Napa Valley, courtesy of Michael Zumpano. I'd come across the *Underground Steroid Handbook* while writing an earlier book and wanted to speak to him for the history I was about to start. Not quite sure what to expect, I found a storyteller who was brimming with anecdotes. He wore several hats for this project—tour guide, sounding board, archivist, and magician who helped to bring Dan Duchaine back to life. This project owes a special debt to his patience and foresight, not to mention his taste in Merlot.

Dan had horribly destructive relationships with women, and two of them—Mary Lou and Shelley Harvey—had harrowing stories to tell. That they told them with such raw honesty, so that the portrayal I have rendered would be complete, is remarkable. Thanks, as well, to Dan's other friends: John Romano, Bruce Kneller, Patrick Arnold, Will Brink, Stan Antosh, Shelley Hominuk, and Nancee Schwartz. Thanks also to Sheila Butch for sharing invaluable bits of family history, some of which even Dan's closest friends did not know.

Dennis Degan has forgotten more about prosecuting steroid cases than most people can remember. Phil Halpern, the Assistant U.S. Attorney in San Diego, calls him "the greatest investigator I've ever known." Perhaps this book will give Dennis some of the credit he is due.

Credit is not a problem for Don Catlin. After he broke the BALCO case open, the head of the Olympic Analytical lab at UCLA became a bona fide media celebrity. Now, one of the great first acts in American life is giving way to a second, thanks to his decision to open a new research center in Los Angeles. As he works on inventing new drug tests (alongside tireless aides such as Caroline Hatton), Don will continue to be a leader in the fight for good sportsmanship and good health.

I wish Terry Madden, the outgoing head of USADA, could have said more. His agency continues to be plagued by the perception that it is too hypersecret. But this book is better for his insights about how he struggled to find his footing in his early years as its leader.

The Dietary Supplement Health and Education Act of 1994 was a profoundly flawed piece of legislation that opened the floodgates to all sorts of mischief. Even so, Loren Israelsen, the lobbyist who worked hard on its passage, believed he was fighting for the rights of the individual consumer. He enriched the section on DSHEA, as did William Schultz, Marcia Lee Taylor, William Llewellyn, Rick Collins, Gary Dykstra, Anthony Almada, Scott Bass, and Phil Schiliro.

Sources on both sides of the law were indispensable to my education. Those in law enforcement include the pseudonymous Jack MacGregor, Dan Simmons, and Rusty Payne at the DEA; Greg Stejskal and Bill Randall, former special agents with the FBI; Phil Halpern of the U.S. Attorney's Office in San Diego; and several others who asked not to be named. Those who ushered me through the steroid underground included Charlie Francis, Victor Conte, Nancee Schwartz, and even more people who asked not to be identified.

Some wonderful writers have covered material included in this book, but I feel especially indebted to a Murderer's Row of colleagues from *ESPN The Magazine:* Luke Cyphers, Tom Farrey,

Amy K. Nelson, and Peter Keating.

All of this would have been a hopeless mess if not for Chris Raymond and Michael Solomon of ESPN Books. Several proposals for this book went nowhere. Chris encouraged me to keep shaping it until I got it right. Once I got a green light, Michael put the book squarely on his shoulders. He was able to see the finished version long before I could. I can't remember one argument, or one day where he wasn't disarmingly calm and enthusiastic. Simply astounding.

Working alongside Michael is a terrific team at ESPN Books: Sandy DeShong, John Glenn, Jessica Welke, and Ellie Seifert. Making it all mesh: Gary Hoenig, the general manager of ESPN Publishing, whose advice is the best in the business.

If any fact is incorrect, the blame is entirely mine. That is because a crack team of research professionals put a ridiculous amount of time into shoring up the manuscript. Anna Katherine Clemmons and Kate Macmillan helped the indefatigable Simon Brennan comb through every word. I can't say enough about Simon's passion and patience. I am also grateful for copy editor Marcella Durand. Thanks as well to David "The Knife" Korzenik for legally vetting everything except this sentence.

Acknowledgments usually end with family members for a reason. At the end of the day, after all of the above people caused me to get way too high or way too low, two people smoothed out the edges. Ellen, my wife, and Jake, my son, kept me on the rails when the train looked a little shaky. The trip with them is always ... well, a trip.

— New York, August 2007

SELECTED BIBLIOGRAPHY

Arnoldi, Katie. *Chemical Pink: A Novel of Obsession.* Forge Books, 2001.

Assael, Shaun, and Mike Mooneyham. *Sex, Lies, and Headlocks: The Real Story of Vince McMahon and World Wrestling Entertainment.* Crown, 2002.

Bahrke, Michael S., and Charles E. Yesalis. *Performance-Enhancing Substances in Sport and Exercise.* Human Kinetics, 2002.

Bryant, Howard. *Juicing the Game: Drugs, Power, and the Fight for the Soul of Major League Baseball.* Viking Press, 2005.

Bass, I. Scott, and Anthony L. Young. *Dietary Supplement Health and Education Act: A Legislative History and Analysis.* The Food and Drug Law Institute, 1996.

Canseco, Jose. *Juiced: Wild Times, Rampant 'Roids, Smash Hits, and How Baseball Got Big.* Regan Books, 2005.

Collins, Rick. *Legal Muscle: Anabolics in America.* Legal Muscle Publishing, 2002.

Courson, Steve, and Lee R. Schreiber. *False Glory: Steelers and Steroids: The Steve Courson Story.* Longmeadow Press, 1991.

Donati, Alessandro. *World Traffic in Doping Substances.* The World Anti-Doping Agency, February 2007.

Dubin, The Honourable Charles L. *Commission of Inquiry into the Use of Drugs and Banned Practices Intended to Increase Athletic Performance.* Canada, 1990.

Duchaine, Dan, and Michael Zumpano. *Underground Steroid Handbook for Men and Women,* OEM Publishing, 1982.

Fainaru-Wada, Mark, and Lance Williams. *Game of Shadows: Barry Bonds, BALCO, and the Steroids Scandal that Rocked Professional Sports.* Gotham Books, 2006.

Fair, John D. *Muscletown USA: Bob Hoffman and the Manly Culture of York Barbell.* Pennsylvania State University Press, 1999.

Francis, Charlie, with Jeff Coplon. *Speed Trap: Inside the Biggest Scandal in Olympic History.* Lester & Orpen Dennys Limited, 1990.

Goldman, Bob, with Patricia J. Bush and Ronald Klatz. *Death in the Locker Room: Steroids & Sports.* Icarus Press, 1984.

Huizenga, Rob. *You're Okay, It's Just a Bruise: A Doctor's Sideline Secrets about Pro Football's Most Outrageous Team.* St. Martin's Griffin, 1994.

Hurley, Dan. *Natural Causes: Death, Lies & Politics in America's Vitamin and Herbal Supplement Industry.* Broadway Books, 2006.

Kolata, Gina. *Ultimate Fitness: The Quest for Truth about Exercise and Health.* Farrar, Straus and Giroux, 2003.

Leigh, Wendy. *Arnold: An Unauthorized Biography.* Congdon & Weed, 1990.

Llewellyn, William. *Anabolics.* 6th ed. Body of Science, 2007.

Mathews, Joe. *The People's Machine: Arnold Schwarzenegger and the Rise of Blockbuster Democracy.* PublicAffairs Books, 2006.

Pope, Jr., Harrison G., Katharine A. Phillips, and Roberto Olivardia. *The Adonis Complex: The Secret Crisis of Male Body Obsession.* The Free Press, 2000.

Pound, Dick. *Inside the Olympics.* John Wiley & Sons, 2004.

Romanowski, Bill, with Adam Schefter and Phil Towle. *Romo: My Life on the Edge: Living Dreams and Slaying Dragons.* William Morrow, 2005.

Shilts, Randy. *And the Band Played On: Politics, People and the AIDS Epidemic.* St. Martin's Press, 1987.

Ungerleider, Steven. *Faust's Gold: Inside the East German Doping Machine.* St. Martin's Press, 2001.

Voet, Willy. *Breaking the Chain: Drugs and Cycling: The True Story.* Yellow Jersey Press, 2002.

U.S. Senate Committee on the Judiciary. *Steroids in Amateur and Professional Sports—The Medical and Social Costs of Steroid Abuse.* U.S. Government Printing Office, 1990.

Wadler, Gary I., and Brian Hainline, MD. *Drugs and the Athlete.* F. A. Davis, 1989.

SOURCE NOTES

INTRODUCTION

Pushed the limits of his school's dress code: Author interview with childhood friend Dana Bourgeois; also high school yearbook photo.

Studying drama at Boston University: "A Guru Who Spreads the Gospel of Steroids," *The New York Times*, November 19, 1988.

Bike shop in Maine: Interview with Bourgeois.

Then he sold the information: All details otherwise not noted from author interview with Michael Zumpano.

"We're going to tell you how": *Underground Steroid Handbook for Men and Women.*

CHAPTER ONE

Dennis Degan tacked the article: All details otherwise not noted from author interview with Dennis Degan.

Fitton pleaded guilty: "British Weightlifter Arrested Following Five Month Chase," The Associated Press, August 26, 1985. Author interview with Phillip Halpern.

The *Sports Illustrated* article: "Steroid Justice," *Sports Illustrated*, December 9, 1985.

Selling on the street: Author interview with William Dillon.

Dillon came up with the idea: "Confessions of a Steroid Smuggler," *Los Angeles Times Magazine*, April 24, 1988.

He bought a stake: Interview with Dillon.

A morphine substitute: http://www.drugs.com/PDR/Nubain_Injection.html.

Three letters on his knuckles: Interview with Dillon.

As soon as they left: Ibid.

If it gets nasty, you won't be good at it: Ibid.

After he was charged: "Sports News," The Associated Press, June 19, 1987; The Associated Press, December 1, 1987.

Could Mansen help out: All details on the case not otherwise noted: "Confessions of a Steroid Smuggler," *Los Angeles Times Magazine*, April 24, 1988.

20 valiums a day and Halcion, too: Interview with Zumpano.

"I've been on edge": "The Unwitting Confessions of a Smuggler," *Los Angeles Times*, October 16, 1988.

CHAPTER TWO

A New Englander who had received: "The Awful Truth About Drugs In Sports," *Outside*, July, 2005.

Catching a late-night flight: "Drugs mar Pan-Am Games," *Christian Science Monitor*, August, 19, 1987; *The Steroids Game: An Expert's Inside Look at Anabolic Steroid use in Sports*, by Charles E. Yesalis and Virginia S. Cowart, pp.181-182; author interview with Don Catlin.

It wasn't until Wednesday: Interview with Don Catlin.

The Games had surpassed *Roots*: "Western White House; How Reagan Spent His Vacation," *The New York Times*, August 15, 1984.

To the senior citizens: Author interviews with Bill March and John D. Fair; also *Muscletown USA: Bob Hoffman and the Manly Culture of York Barbell*, by John D. Fair.

His exploits were breathlessly reported: *Strength & Health* magazine, July 1962.

"Then I guess we can't": *Speed Trap: Inside the Biggest Scandal in Olympic History*, by Charlie Francis with Jeff Coplon, p. 206. Author interview with Charlie Francis.

But everywhere else in the track world: Ibid., p. 103.

Next, Francis brought the list: Commission of Inquiry into the Use of Drugs and Banned Practices Intended to Increase Athletic Performance, Charles Dubin, Commissioner; Ben Johnson's testimony, p. 282.

He failed to beat Lewis: *Speed Trap*, pp. 139-140.

His Toronto contact suggested: Ibid., p. 162. Interview with Francis.

"And it would only be afterward": "Bursting From the Shadows," *Sports Illustrated*, November 30, 1987.

Fearing a lawsuit: "U.S. track stars take cheap shots at Big Ben," *The Toronto Star*, December 15, 1987; "Johnson 'shocked' by Lewis drug hints," *The Toronto Star*, September 6, 1987.

"If I was losing": Ibid, September 6, 1987.

He had told another Canadian Olympian: Dubin Commission, p. 198.

It merely asked that Francis: Ibid., p. 205.

The next day: "Big Ben, coach must reconcile or gold is lost," *The Toronto Star*, June 28, 1988.

Astaphan was also nervous enough: Dubin Commission, pp. 297-299.

There was just one more formality: Ibid., p. 285.

"My skin is getting so tight": "Diary noted every dose; top sprinter sought perfect diet of drugs inquiry told," *The Toronto Star*, March 14, 1989.

He revealed that he had been operating: Dubin Commission, p. 210.

CHAPTER THREE

The bleached landscape: ludb.clui.org/ex/i/CA4983. Interview with Halpern.

A box of hand grenades: Author interview with Dan Duchaine's defense attorney, Nancee Schwartz.

Instead, Duchaine went in the opposite direction: February 27,

1989, Duchaine letter to Sheila Butch.

The cops who were shadowing him: Interview with Nancee Schwartz, November 2005.

Women's bodybuilding didn't coalesce: Author interview with female bodybuilding historians Steve Wennerstrom and Bill Dobbins, February 2006.

When Robert Mapplethorpe: www.iol.ie/~webfoto/maple7j.htm.

Her successor, Corey Everson: www.bodyshaping.com/swimsuitgallery/coreyeverson.htm.

"It's Glucophage," he said: Author interview with Sandra Blackie; www.healthsquare.com/newrx/GLU1188.htm.

After Duchaine married: http://sandgate.co.clark.nv.us/servlet/RecMarriage.

"The girls know each other": February 27, 1989, letter to Sheila Butch.

In September 1988: "Sure, Oprah slimmed down fast, but liquid diets aren't right for everyone," *Chicago Tribune,* December 28, 1988.

The product's manufacturer: "Dieters Seek Drink That Made Grand Oprah Into Light Oprah," *Business First-Columbus,* December 12, 1988.

The ratings were the highest: "Oprah's Diet Show Scores Record High Numbers," *PR Newswire,* November 16, 1988.

Newsweek **declared:** "Oprah: Profile in Curvage," *Newsweek,* November 28, 1988.

Initially, its publisher: Author interview with Jason Mathas.

A call was set up: All details of the family come from Duchaine's sisters, Sheila Butch and Elaine Lanning.

This was before he went: http://www.everybody.co.nz/page-c061d5bb-1ca6-47a9-8d89-6a12d12c128b.aspx.

U.S. Customs officials had been pressuring: Background interview with United States Customs agent, November 2005. Also, brief author interview with Juan Macklis.

So long as he stayed outside: The timing is inexact. Press reports dated October 13, 1989 ("U.S. Paid $1 Million to Insurgents, Noriega Says," *St. Louis Post-Dispatch*") state the deal was consummated two and a half years before, or roughly May 1987. The indictment against Duchaine, William Dillon and David Jenkins was filed on May 20, 1987.

A year earlier: "U.S. Paid $1 Million to Insurgents, Noriega Says," *St. Louis Post-Dispatch*, October 13, 1989.

Since the deal had been struck: Ibid.; "Noriega Linked to Steroid Smuggling, Mexico Says," *The New York Times*, December 3, 1989.

And shortly after his captors released him: "U.S. Athletes Advised: Get Your Steroids Here!" *The New York Times*, September 25, 1989.

Ronald Reagan promptly signed: *Legal Muscle*, by Rick Collins, p. 5.

"My answer has been simple": "Steroids in Amateur and Professional Sports—The Medical and Social Costs of Steroid Abuse," transcript of Senate hearings, April 3, 1989 and May 9, 1989, p. 101.

The Department of Health: *Legal Muscle* p. 5.

Moreover, they can be safely used: Senate Hearings, p. 71.

"I tell them to drop": Ibid., pp. 12, 42.

CHAPTER FOUR

Lyle Alzado parked his Rolls-Royce: Address provided by Accurint.com.

He hated the mechanics of television: Transcript of unedited interview with Kris Alzado for ESPN Classic, October 24, 2002.

He went back to his buddies: "Big Night," *ESPN The Magazine*, January 21, 2003.

It was the kind of pause: Published reports and author interview with Janice Alzado, January 2, 2006.

Courson testified: "U.S. Senate told of NFL Use; Drugs in Sport," *The Times* (London), May 11, 1989.

When it came time: Transcript of unedited interview with Marc Lyons for ESPN Classic, May 21, 2003. Author interview with Lyons.

He ate yeast pills: Transcript of unedited interview with Howie Long for ESPN Classic, May 21, 2003.

Any time, the school's football team: Transcript of unedited interview with Dave Downey for ESPN Classic, September 21, 2002.

Then Alzado sped away: Lyons interview, May 21, 2003.

But he was taking so many drugs: "I'm Sick and I'm Scared," *Sports Illustrated*, July 8, 1991.

His body was working: Ibid.

"Dad asked me for money": Author interview with Janice Alzado, January 12, 2006.

He was on Equipoise: Ibid.

Attendance in the NFL: "The face of sweeping change," *Sports Illustrated*, September 10, 1990.

Last year alone, the league had suspended: "The NFL Fails Its Drug Test," *Sports Illustrated*, July 10, 1989.

Rozelle announced: "N.F.L. Bans 15 for Drugs or Steroids," *The New York Times*, August 30, 1989.

It ran below a headline: "Sportsline," *USA Today*, November 2, 1989.

As inmate No.: Federal Bureau of prisons web site locator: http://www.bop.gov/iloc2/LocateInmate.jsp.

The time went mercifully: Author interview with John Romano.

Thanks to the efforts of Senator Joe Biden: *Legal Muscle*, p. 10.

In prison, Duchaine had developed: Interview with Romano.

Soon after, Kris filed for divorce: Interview with Janice Alzado, January 12, 2006.

Shelley Smith was no novice: Author interview with Shelley Smith.

"The publicity generated": Coming Soon, Alzado the Sequel," *Sports Illustrated*, July 2, 1990.

"I'm clean": Taken from video of *Cutting Edge with Maria Shriver*, NBC.

In fact, he was taking a drug: Author interview with Kathy Alzado Murray.

The government used human cadavers: http://arbl.cvmbs. colostate.edu/hbooks/pathphys/endocrine/hypopit/gh.html.

After recipients: www.medicalnewstoday.com/medicalnews. php?newsid=7194; www.nih.gov/news/pr/apr2004/nichd-07.htm.

The April 1990 issue: "Growth Hormone: Does It Really Increase Lean Mass and Decrease Fat?" *Muscle & Fitness*, April 1990.

He also began taking: http://www.testosterones.com/cypionate. htm.

He'd just take it easy: "Alzado Strains A Calf Muscle," *Los Angeles Times*, July 17, 1990.

When the team left: "Davis' quandary not only problem; Raiders' questions outnumber answers," *The Orange County Register*, July 29, 1990.

He ran it back 15 yards: "Defense Fuels Raiders Past Bears, 20-3," *Los Angeles Times*, August 25, 1990.

The three were walking down Melrose: Author interview with Cindy Alzado.

CHAPTER FIVE

Mornings would begin: Interview with Romano.

Muscle magazines reflected it: *MuscleMag International*, November, 1991; *Ironman*, May, 1991; *Ironman*, September, 1991.

The 27-year-old had grown up in the heart: Author interview with Shelley Harvey.

Since its structure is similar: "Drug Story," *SF Weekly*, November 29, 1995.

A video of his experiment: The video was provided to the author by the not-for-profit Project GHB.

The researcher concluded: USA v. Wood, p. 356.

Knowing a good sales pitch: *SF Weekly*, November 29, 1995.

There was initially some question: "Survivors, officials square off over dead woman's frozen head," *The Orange County Register*, January, 18, 1988; "Coroners baffled by bizarre mystery of the frozen head," *The Courier Mail*, January, 26, 1988.

"Jesus, Larry," Dan said: Author interview with Larry Wood.

She was a bit irked: Section based on interview with Alzado Murray.

Others had labels from East Germany: There is some discrepancy over when this happened. Alzado Murray tells the story this way. In his book, *You're Okay, It's Just A Bruise: A Doctor's Sideline Secrets about Pro Football's Most Outrageous Team*, Rob Huizenga recalls the search happening later, when Lyle was away for a radiation treatment. The assortment of pills comes from Huizenga's book, p. 290.

In November 1990: *SF Weekly*, November 29, 1995.

Undaunted, the chemist simply moved his lab: Author interview with Eugene Thirolf, director of the Department of Justice's Office of Consumer Litigation.

And on December 13: USA v. Lawrence Wood and Daniel Duchaine, p. 87.

"I'll have him call you": USA v. Wood, p. 87-90; the pre-sentence report confirms the 2/20 call.

After a workout and breakfast: The court record says that he rented the box on March 6, under the name Carolyn Rasmus.

Roughly the size of a large bedroom: Description recalled by Zumpano, who visited the site.

"I can't play at that size": Author interview with Rob Huizenga.

Then he switched: *You're Okay, It's Just A Bruise: A Doctor's Sideline Secrets about Pro Football's Most Outrageous Team*, by Rob Huizenga, p. 285.

"Well, Lyle, there's something": Ibid., p. 286.

"Lyle Alzado, an imposing former": "110-Pound Deputy Marshal More Than A Match For Alzado," *Los Angeles Times*, April 17, 1991.

CHAPTER SIX

"I'm really sorry, Shelley": Interview with Harvey.

"They think they can fuck with me": Interview with Romano.

A few months earlier, he had been in a mall: Interview with Alzado Murray.

It ranged from grand jury testimony: Interview with Degan.

It was the largest such operation: "Sting Operation Nabs Iranian Counterfeit Drug Dealer," *FDA Consumer*, April 1989.

Congress enacted the bill: "Cracking down on Controlled Substance," *St. Louis Post-Dispatch*, June 23, 1991.

The accompanying story: "Hulk: Bulk from a bottle?" *USA Today*, June 20, 1991.

Fortunately, he had found an outlet: Section adapted from *Sex, Lies & Headlocks: The Real Story of Vince McMahon and World Wrestling Entertainment*, by Shaun Assael & Mike Mooneyham, pp. 86-95; additional information from Degan.

Hogan got his chance: http://www.imdb.com/title/tt0084602/trivia.

"The most important thing": *CBS This Morning* transcript, July 8, 1991.

As Dave Kehr noted: "Terminating a trend?" *Chicago Tribune*, July 3, 1991.

"Then in the afternoons": Transcript of *Larry King Live*, June 27, 1991.

Before he lost consciousness: This scene is pasted together from the recollections of several sources, none of who could remember all of the details, including Harvey. A police report on the accident could not be found.

"If you were, you'd forgive me": Recollection of Romano.

CHAPTER SEVEN

Thanks to the two strokes: November 5, 1992 Letter to Sheila Butch.

"But you will hear testimony": USA v. Wood, pp. 61-62.

But "what this case will not show": Ibid., p. 67.

"Vitamins aren't regulated": Ibid., p. 553.

"GHB and LSD produce": Ibid., p. 346.

"Secondly, is the fact": Ibid., p. 354.

***Time* magazine had recently profiled him:** *Time*, November 4, 1991.

"It's a sedative drug": USA v. Wood, p. 446.

"You know, animals can't tell you": Ibid., pp. 448-451, 456.

Since he could no longer speak: Interview with Alzado Murray.

His manager had rented a ballroom: Huizenga, pp. 303-305.

His once-booming voice: Author interview with Derrick Barton.

Then, staring at his wife: The Associated Press, March 24, 1992; interview with Alzado Murray.

Their destination was her family home: Author Interview Ed Davis.

As his latest movie: "This Sequel's A Real Killer," *Herald Sun*, March 19, 1992.

CHAPTER EIGHT

When the clinic was secured: "Armed Agents Make 'B-Vitamin Bust' in Kent," *Seattle Post-Intelligencer*, May 7, 1992.

With his soft Midwestern cadence: Author interview with Loren Israelsen.

And, as Israelsen argued: "FDA: Vitamin Claims Must Be Backed Up," *Los Angeles Times*, December 30, 1993.

Recognizing that the law was imperfect: *Dietary Supplement Health and Education Act: A Legislative History and Analysis*, by I. Scott Bass & Anthony L. Young, p. 15.

The FDA's internal analysis: "FDA: Vitamin Claims Must Be Backed Up," *Los Angeles Times*, December 30, 1993.

"If you don't like the rules": Interview with Israelsen. The official he said he was speaking with, then-deputy commissioner for policy, Michael Taylor, declined to be interviewed.

"I can't even express": "Clinic Operator Baffled, Outraged," *The Seattle Times*, May 8, 1992.

He had even sold vitamins: "Scorin' with Orrin; Orrin Hatch, U.S. senator," *Washington Monthly*, September 1, 2001.

And considering the small stake: "Strange Bedfellows Fight For An Unlikely Powerlobby on Capitol Hill," *States News Service*, September 29, 1994.

Grandly labeled the Health Freedom Act: "F.D.A. Steps Up Effort to Control Vitamin Claims," *The New York Times*, August 9, 1992.

Representative Henry Waxman: Ibid.

When that didn't pan out: "Mr. Big," *Outside*, September 2003.

The burgeoning minimogul: http://www.answers.com/topic/bill-phillips-author; ad from p. 131, *MuscleMag International*, August 1992.

The editor's note in his second issue: "No Holds Barred," *Muscle Media 2000*, Summer 1992.

Phillips was sure he could sell: "Survival of the Fittest," *Denver Westword*, November 15, 2001.

He also put Connelly: Ibid.

As former A's DH: Author Interview with Dave Parker.

McGwire had grown up: *Juicing the Game: Drugs, Power, and the Fight for the Soul of Major League Baseball*, by Howard Bryant, p. 117.

It often looked like the backstage area: "Who Knew?" *ESPN The Magazine*, November 21, 2005.

Dumping Canseco now: "Texas-sized Trade," *Sports Illustrated*, September 14, 1992.

A personal trainer: "Hitting the Mark" *Daily News* (New York), March 13, 2005.

He lived with, and worked for: "Reggie Still Has Impact, *Capital Times*, June 11, 1992.

Besides training Jackson: "Jax upset his name was dragged in," *Newsday*, March 14, 2005; beeper store detail from author interview with Curtis Wenzlaff.

Notes that he showed: "Hitting the Mark," *Daily News* (New York), March 13, 1992.

Hours before the A's: "A's 'Little Lineup' Sputters in Loss," *San Francisco Chronicle*, July 8, 1992.

Dan Duchaine didn't want his girlfriend: Interview with Harvey.

"This is a *real* marriage": October 23, 1992 letter to Sheila Butch.

"We're planning to extract": September 27, 1992 letter to Sheila Butch.

At four in the morning: http://bphc.hrsa.gov/nhdp.

"All the inmates are either sick:" October 27, 1992 letter to Sheila Butch.

As he told his sister: November 5, 1992 letter to Sheila Butch.

Walk around, shake some hands: Author interview with Alan Hoeting, former director, FDA Office of Enforcement.

He asked Halpern: Interview with Halpern.

Dykstra decided to give his speech: Author interview with Gary Dykstra.

Standing before the Senate: *Dietary Supplement Health and Education Act: A Legislative History and Analysis*, p. 23.

The Council for Responsible Nutrition: Author interview with Dr. Annette Dickenson, former CRN president; also Dr. John Hathcock, CRN Vice President, Scientific & International Affairs.

One, a tough-talking New Yorker: Author interview with Gerry Kessler.

CHAPTER NINE

He had also helped: "'Engineered food' pumps up firm," *Rocky Mountain News*, March 2, 1994.

Phillips had turned himself: "No Holes Barred," *Muscle Media*, December-January 1994.

Not everyone thought Met-Rx: Author interview with John "Kim" Wood.

Using the tough new steroid laws: "While preparing for the Super Bowl, some members of the Dallas Cowboys are just as concerned with winning as making sports drug free," *Business Wire*, January 25, 1994.

The same issue: *Muscle Media*, June-July 1994.

Byrd was especially so: "Two Bay Area Men Are Indicted In Sale of Steroids," *Los Angeles Times*, March 13, 1991; USA v. Byrd, et al. (CR-00102-FMS).

"I really don't think": Author interview with Anthony Almada.

They were coolly designed: Ibid.

The night before, he was part: "Rangers Update," *The Dallas Morning News*, August 11, 1994.

The players were feuding: "La Russa's Work May Be For Naught," *Chicago Tribune*, August 14, 1994.

Casually, he would mention: "Muscling Inside Ring of Steroids," *Daily News* (New York), March 14, 2005; author interview with Greg Stejskal.

Ted Kennedy, once an implacable: *Dietary Supplement Health and Education Act: A Legislative History and Analysis*, p. 29.

Just as important: Ibid., p. 28.

There was still a brick wall: Author interview with William Schultz, former subcommittee counsel to Henry Waxman.

"I want to make very clear": *Dietary Supplement Health and Education Act: A Legislative History and Analysis*, p. 29.

Supplement bill supporters: Author interview with Philip Schiliro, chief of staff to Henry Waxman.

Bill Phillips was calmly anticipating: Interview with Almada.

Almada had to look no further: *Muscle Media*, August-September 1994.

Gold's was up to 400: "Gold's steps in beverage ring," *Advertising Age*, April 12, 1993.

Joe Weider's *Muscle & Fitness*: "The Anatomy of Misleading Ads," *Muscle & Fitness*, May 1994.

"I hope we're not being set up": Author interview with I. Scott Bass, partner at Sidley & Austin, Washington, D.C.

CHAPTER TEN

In September, he had suffered another stroke: Escorted Trip Authorization forms—6/29, 9/21 and 9/30/94—from Dan Duchaine's federal Bureau of Prisons file, obtained under the Freedom of Information Act; www.americanheart.org/presenter.jhtml?identifier=3018935.

In perhaps the ultimate indignity: Work Performance Rating, 8/16-9/15/94, federal Bureau of Prisons file.

"I . . . know . . . exactly": Interview with Romano.

All the time he had spent: This story was told by Duchaine to Zumpano.

"She's not coming": Interview with Romano.

"I've moved on from the old days": Author interview with Sandra Blackie.

"To be blunt": "Ask The Guru," *Muscle Media 2000*, January 1995.

McGwire was visiting Zumpano: Interview with Zumpano.

The brothers looked so much alike: "Great Chase Turns Into Great Debate," *Los Angeles Times*, August 25, 1998.

As reporter Tom Farrey noted: "Desperate for the Winning Edge . . ." *The Seattle Times*, February 6, 1994.

When the professor reported: "Food Supplement Creatine Can Build Muscle, But Risks Unknown," The Associated Press, September 16, 1996; also interview with Almada.

It wasn't long before half the teams: Almada recalled this story, and the material used in the rest of the section.

Kneller was a registered nurse: This section is based entirely on the recollection of Bruce Kneller, except where otherwise noted.

So it shouldn't be any surprise: "Rant," *Muscle Media*, November 1995.

One of his new ideas involved: The product was linked to Duchaine in an Amateur Athletic Foundation newsletter; "Morning Briefing: Don't Forget Incentive Clause For Hitting 60 Or More Homers," *Los Angeles Times*, May 23, 1995.

Broke but having a blast: Government's brief in opposition to Stan Antosh's appeal, filed September 10, 1998, in USA v. Antosh.

Gave him a bottle of GHB: Ibid.

GHB produced a wicked high: Author interview with Stan Antosh.

At the suggestion of one of his customers: Ibid.

Hospitalized for a nervous breakdown: USA v. Antosh.

The person responsible: All details in government's brief in opposition to Stan Antosh's appeal, filed September 10, 1998 in USA v. Antosh.

Pounding his glove in left field: http://www.baseball-almanac.com/teamstats/schedule.php?y=1996&t=OAK.

In an ironic twist, Wenzlaff's part-time employer: "They're Starting to Have A Blast," *The Boston Globe*, May 18, 1996.

McGwire was also on a tear: www.retrosheet.org.

As it happened, the A's lost: American League Game Summaries, *The Sports Network*, May 18, 1996.

"I'll look at the menu": "Giambi and McGwire's Power Lunches," *The Miami Herald*, May 28, 1996; extrapolated.

The 10 pounds of muscle: "Is This Dr. Evil?" *Sports Illustrated*, October 9, 2006. Author interview with Patrick Arnold.

A red Lamborghini: "Looking like a million; At 31, tycoon Bill Phillips rules bodybuilding empire," *Rocky Mountain News*, September 1, 1996; interview with Romano.

CHAPTER ELEVEN

Lausanne, Switzerland, November 28, 1996: "IOC Executive Board to Assess Atlanta's Problems," The Associated Press, October 8, 1996.

He had 16,000 samples: This detail and others from this chapter, interview with Catlin.

By the closing ceremonies: "Two Olympians test positive for steroids," *Milwaukee Journal Sentinel*, August 6, 1996.

But, like the samples he sought: Interview with Catlin and his aide, Caroline Hatton.

"There were several other steroid positives": "Revealed: four more Olympic drug users," *Sunday Times*, November 17, 1996.

It was too new to be trusted: "IOC Throws Out Five Potentially Positive Doping Tests," The Associated Press, November 28, 1996.

San Francisco, California, January 15, 1997: Osmo Invoice No. 852, 1/15/97.

The linebacker who was on his way: "Ex-Raider to face steroid questions," *San Francisco Chronicle*, January 27, 2005.

Even strength coaches got into the act: Author interview with Laura Moore.

Its first cover story: "The Poor Man's Guide To Making GHB," *Dirty Dieting*, March 1997.

In a few years, Arnold would build: Ibid.

His latest relationship: All details about the relationship, except where otherwise noted, are from author interview with "Mary Lou."

His temperature had soared to 103 degrees: Recalled by Romano.

"Better still, stay out of my life": Recalled by Kneller, and also confirmed by Romano, who heard about it from Duchaine.

Divided into neat sections were 500 pills: *Romo: My Life On the Edge: Living Dreams and Slaying Dragons*, by Bill Romanowski with Adam Schefter and Phil Towle, p. 161.

Romo would be "sitting on the steps": "Taking His Medicine," *Sports Illustrated*, May 25, 1998.

A television audience: "Super Bowl Audience is 3rd Largest for TV Show," *St. Louis Post-Dispatch*, January 27, 1998.

As soon as he learned: Author interview with Bill Romanowski; also *Romo*, p. 160.

Giving interviews in EAS gear: "EAS Bulks Up With Creatine, Broncos," *Rocky Mountain News*, June 28, 1998.

"They're winded!": "Davis Delivers, Dashes All Doubts," *The Seattle Times*, January 26, 1998.

In all, it was enough to prepare: "Drug Pedaling," *Sports Illustrated*, July 5, 1999; *Breaking the Chain: Drugs and Cycling: the True Story*, by Willy Voet, pp. 1-10.

His wife also handed over: Ibid.

The Spanish aristocrat: Interview with Catlin; this reflects his expert opinion.

"If it's just the second case": "Samaranch Seeks to Clarify Rules Governing Drug Use," *The Washington Post*, July 27, 1998.

The Bureau of Prisons: U.S. government motion in Antosh case.

"Sitting on the top shelf": "'Andro' pill OK in baseball, not in other sports," The Associated Press, August 22, 1998.

On a visit to Scottsdale: All recollections from "Mary Lou."

As for competitive bodybuilding: http://www.graphicmuscle.com/index.cfm?go2=contests_year&ContestYearID=234.

CHAPTER TWELVE

The IOC was being swallowed: "No medals for the IOC," *Time*, February 15, 1999.

Pound proposed creating: *Inside the Olympics: A Behind-the-Scenes Look at the Politics, the Scandals and the Glory of the Games*, by Dick Pound, pp. 69-71.

His longtime medical advisor: "Oly: IOC struggling not to have drugs summit overwhelmed," AAP Newsfeed, February 2, 1999.

But the Salt Lake scandal: "The Real Scandal," *Newsweek*, February 15, 1999.

"Everyone must know: "More calls for Samaranch to resign as IOC president," *The Vancouver Sun*, February 3, 1999.

A study in the journal *Pediatrics*: "The Real Scandal," *Newsweek*, February 15, 1999.

"We are not a court": "Samaranch calls for 'autonomous' anti-drug agency," The Associated Press, February 2, 1999.

The plan was shot down: "Samaranch Slammed," *The Toronto Sun*, February 3, 1999.

What was left was a six-point "declaration": "Text of the adopted anti-doping declaration," The Associated Press, February 4, 1999.

Flashing a self-satisfied grin: "IOC Comes In For Hard Landing," *Los Angeles Times*, February 5, 1999.

For comfort, Duchaine reached out: Author interview with Shelley Hominuk.

He wrote a living will: Ibid.; also, interview with "Mary Lou."

On Christmas Eve: Recollections of Sheila Butch. At her brother's funeral, Butch spoke with Dan's adoptive Aunt Loraine, who provided her with the other details used in the section.

Shortly before 10 p.m.: San Diego Medical Examiner report, Investigative Narrative.

CHAPTER THIRTEEN

A third of what his Eraser had taken in: http://www.the-movie-times.com/thrsdir/actors/actorProfiles.mv?arnold.

As *Los Angeles Times* writer: *The People's Machine: Arnold Schwarzenegger and the Rise of Blockbuster Democracy*, by Joe Mathews, p. 61.

Beyond that, Schwarzenegger subscribed: Ibid., pp. 54-60, 63.

"I felt that was eventually": Ibid., p. 39.

But most were content: "Women Flex, Flaunt and Strut," *Columbus Dispatch*, March 6, 1999; "Hard Bodies, Hearty Cheers," *Columbus Dispatch*, March 7, 1999; "Schwarzenegger: I'll Be Back at Vets Memorial," *Columbus Dispatch*, March 8, 1999.

Victor Conte, Jr., was born: Details taken from transcript of interview used to write "Last Laugh," *ESPN The Magazine*, December 20, 2004.

One night, a bunch of goons walked in: *In My Father's Name*, by Mark Arax.

Conte studied accounting: "Bay Area lab owner's troubled past; Success coupled with tax difficulties and unraveling family life," *San Francisco Chronicle*, October 26, 2003.

After their separation: "Blood Money," *ESPN The Magazine*, November 10, 2003; "Bay Area lab owner's troubled past; success coupled with tax difficulties and unraveling family life," *San Francisco Chronicle*, October 26, 2003.

Wearing a white lab coat: The year is uncertain. Conte says it was 1996, but Romanowski says it was 1998.

He was awaiting the publication: "North Castle Partners, EAS Announce Equity Partnership," *Business Wire*, September 2, 1999.

After Conte made a long: *Romo: My Life On The Edge*, by Bill Romanowski, p.177.

Arnold's advance made the crystals: Ibid.

One of the more voluble posters: http://groups.google.com/group/misc.fitness.weights/browse_thread/thread/854a2f185d8cdf94/847c84d42aa95e81?lnk=st&q=misc.fitness.weights+Victor+Conte&rnum=4&hl=en#847c84d42aa95e81.

"I have something": Interview with Arnold.

In a 1995 post: http://groups.google.com/group/misc.fitness. weights/browse_thread/thread/38f11689f6739697/751280366ffae86 e?lnk=st&q=Patrick+Arnold+MT%27s+androgenic+potency&rnum=1 #751280366ffae86e.

Then, Freeman literally walked on water: "Greatest Show on Earth," *Sports Illustrated*, October 18, 2000.

Gloating to *The New York Times*: "2000 Sydney Games; At Long Last, Her Golden Moment," *The New York Times*, September 11, 2000.

In a flurry of secret meetings: This comes from a source with knowledge of the negotiations.

Four days before: "Hunter Unable to Compete In Games," *Chicago Tribune*, September 12, 2000.

On a chilly, drizzly Saturday: "Sydney 2000: Track and Field; Golden Redemption for Jones and Greene," *The New York Times*, September 24, 2000; "Marion Takes to the Air," *Newsweek*, October 2, 2000.

Famed attorney Johnnie Cochran: "Jones could be a guiding light in Sydney," *Tampa Tribune*, July 9, 2000.

Montgomery was once: "Nowhere to Run," *ESPN The Magazine*, June 27, 2004.

A couple of weeks earlier: The timing here is as follows: The Olympic trials were held in late July. Conte recalled getting the call from Gaines in the first week of August. *Game of Shadows* reports the episode differently, saying that it was another sprinter, Alvin Harrison, who tipped Montgomery to Contein the summer of 2000.

Don Catlin was just settling into a seat: "Sob story as told by a downright mean and innocent man," *The Australian*, September 27, 2000.

Then she begged the press: "The Olympics Day 12; He failed 4 drug tests but says: I'm innocent," *The Advertiser*, September 27, 2000.

Ten days later, a stunned Gore: "GOP Raises Ruckus Over Wayward Chad;" "Enlisted Ranks Could Hold Key to Florida Results," *San Francisco Chronicle*, November 17, 2000.

Tim Montgomery, meanwhile: This article is from an Associated Press story that ran on page 5 of the *San Francisco Chronicle* on

November 17, the same day Conte said the meeting occurred. In "Nowhere to Run," (*ESPN The Magazine*) the date as listed as mid-November. In *Game of Shadows*, p. 95, the date is listed as "six weeks after the closing ceremonies in Sydney."

An improved drug that would take them: This refers to THG, which Arnold sent Conte for the first time on February 9, 2001.

CHAPTER FOURTEEN

Precisely one year earlier: All background details from author interview with Terry Madden.

As the report concluded: "Report of the USOC Select Task Force on Drug Externalization," December 3, 1999, p. 1.

He added to the drama: Author interview with Wade Exum; also "USOC Drug chief resigns, alleges 'hostile, racist'" The Associated Press, June 14, 2000.

White House drug czar: "Doctors Say USOC Allowed Doping to Go Unchallenged," *Salt Lake Tribune*, August 28, 2000.

It was a dizzying baptism: From USADA press release: 163 in 4QW 2000 and 156 in 1Q 2001. In competition tests were 295 in 4Q 2000 and 896 were in competition in 1Q 2001.

It was an overachieving 16-year-old: Personal details from author interview with Lynn Jacobson, father of Raelyn Jacobson.

At the U.S. Fencing Junior Olympics in February: http://www. usantidoping.org/files/active/resources/press_releases/PressRelease_ 5_1_2001.pdf

Braves manager Bobby Cox: "Giant 6, Braves 3," The Associated Press, May 20, 2001; "Brilliant Bonds not enough," *San Francisco Chronicle*, May 21, 2001.

In the fall of 2000: *Game of Shadows*, p. 113.

It was reissued six years later: http://sports.espn.go.com/espn/ eticket/story?page=steroidsExc&num=19

Tu Mingde was in a surprisingly good mood: "Beijing Wins Bid for 2008 Olympic Games," *The New York Times*, July 14, 2001.

According to a report issued by Amnesty International: Ibid.

Though Catlin couldn't prove it: Interview with Catlin.

Because China had little history: "Synchronized Winning," *Observer Sport Monthly*, October 1, 2006.

Crediting exotic supplements: Ibid.

He Huixian, a spokesman, announced: "Chinese Withdraw 6 Runners And Coach," *The New York Times*, September 7, 2000.

From his lab in Champaign: Affidavit in support of warrant to search the home and workplace of Patrick Arnold, pp. 21-22.

Most of all, his spirit: "McGwire's right knee was getting stronger," *St. Louis Post-Dispatch*, November 14, 2001.

La Russa sized up his slugger: "Cards fall in Round 1," *St. Louis Post-Dispatch*, October 15, 2001.

Despite his warm words: "Just the Fax, Mac?" *St. Louis Post-Dispatch*, November 13, 2001.

CHAPTER FIFTEEN

In Spain, where it was marketed: "Killy warned IOC on darbepoetin," *Agence France Presse*, February 25, 2002.

Out of 300 samples: "Amid Progress, Drug-Testing Still Produces Mixed Results," *The Washington Post*, March 20, 2002.

And while it took seven months: Ibid.; interview with Catlin.

He had won two medals: "Muehlegg Wins Second Gold," *The New York Times*, February 15, 2002.

Things were going so well for him: "Drug busters; Anti-doping sleuths finding new ways to put the squeeze on juiced athletes," Copley News Service, November 5, 2003.

"I think you should see this": Interview with Hatton.

The U.S. Olympic training center: http://www.chulavistaconvis.org/olympic.asp.

A sport in which riders travel: Ibid; http://www.velodromes.com/peking.html.

At their showdown: "Legalities impede speedskater's bid for Olympic cycling sport," The Associated Press, August 20, 2000.

When Witty boycotted the event: Ibid.

The win was overturned: "Speedskater will ride in Sydney for American cycling team," The Associated Press, August 25, 2000.

The two biked regularly: Author interview with Tammy Thomas.

Catlin turned up a signature that resembled: "Drug Testers Have Designs on New Steroid," *The Washington Post*, March 8, 2003.

And Patrick Arnold's own posts: Ibid.; American Arbitration Association decision, USADA v. Tammy Thomas, p. 6.

"Thank you for your time": Interview with Catlin.

Cali, Columbia, June 23, 2002: Notification date comes from USADA.

Her comeback was all but complete: "Cycling must stop back pedaling on drug use," *Morning Call* (Allentown, Penn.), July 10, 2002.

It was from the U.S. Anti-Doping Agency: Interview with Thomas.

"Needless to say, if you know anyone": Arnold search warrant affidavit, p. 28.

In an official reply: USADA v. Thomas, p. 252.

CHAPTER SIXTEEN

The Panthers were faced with the prospect: "Panthers Cut Longtime Star," *Charlotte Observer*, February 27, 2003.

Over the past six months: Wadler report, Exhibit in USA v. James Shortt; "Medical records of ex-Panthers reveal ill effects, multiple refills leading to Super Bowl," *Charlotte Observer*, August 27, 2006.

A third, center Jeff Mitchell: Wadler report, USA v. James Shortt, p.10.

The NFL, however, considered it a steroid: http://skepdic.com/dhea.html; http://www.quackwatch.org/01QuackeryRelatedTopics/dhea.html.

"They're not going to want to do that": Transcript, pp. 1-8, Government's Docket Document 41-2, USA v. James Shortt.

Then shock set in: Author interview with Orioles team doctor, William Goldiner.

He remembered Bechler brooding: "Senator, His Son Get Boosts From Makers of Ephedra," *Los Angeles Times*, March 5, 2003.

A few months later, the legislation: Author interview with Marcia Lee Taylor, Partnership for a Drug-Free America.

It also showed how the senator's son: "Senator, His Son Get Boosts From Makers of Ephedra," *Los Angeles Times*, March 5, 2003.

During a barnstorming tour of Japan: Author interview with Bobby Alejo, formerly Jason Giambi's personal trainer.

Bonds, meanwhile, introduced his trainer: *Game of Shadows*, p. 131.

"I'd sure like to prove it": "The exclusive inside story of the Balco steroids investigation and the government's attempt to bring down Barry Bonds," *Playboy*, May 1, 2004.

On this night, White was aroused from his sleep: Ibid.

In other words, by slightly changing: Description from Hatton.

It behaved exactly the way Catlin predicted: "Discovering a Steroid (The Baboon Was Key)," *The Mercury News*, July 29, 2004.

After all, Schwarzenegger was so friendly: *The People's Machine*, p. 139.

Two years earlier, the *National Enquirer*: "His Media Muscle Has Gone Flabby," *Los Angeles Times*, July 10, 2005.

"We're not going to pull up any dirt": "Muscle Mentor Keeps Tabs on Ah-nold," *Daily News* (New York), August 20, 2003.

Pecker told Schwarzenegger: "Anatomy of a governor's media deal; how Schwarzenegger and publisher decided to help one another," *The International Herald Tribune*, July 19, 2005.

It was his first inkling: Author interview with Victor Conte.

"He's going down": "Blood Money," *ESPN The Magazine*, November 10, 2003

This much is clear: IRS Memorandum of Conte interview, September 3, 2003.

Steroids were so far down the list: Email from Louis Reedt, U.S. Sentencing Commission, to Tom Farrey, March 28, 2006.

CHAPTER SEVENTEEN

"It's a conspiracy involving chemists": The author was on the conference call; also http://espn.go.com/oly/news/2003/1016/1639608.html.

Madden had taken the story: "Grand jury probes nutrient company; Burlingame firm boasts of ties to star athletes," *San Francisco Chronicle*, October 14, 2003.

Made it front-page news: From author's notes of the press conference.

The latest poster boy: "Banned Swimmer Wins Case Over Supplements," The Associated Press, May 14, 2005.

"There's going to be a little something": Interview with Madden.

"By bringing hope to the oppressed": President's State of the Union Message to Congress and the Nation," *The New York Times*, January 21, 2004.

A half hour later: "Bush, Somber and Determined, Stresses War Against Terror," *The New York Times*, January 21, 2004.

The United States hadn't pursued: Author interview with Jack "MacGregor."

The U.S. Attorney General, John Ashcroft: "Indictments Put Baseball, Other Sports In Tenuous Spot," *The Washington Post*, February 13, 2004.

When Novitzky's agents finally left: US v. Comprehensive Drug Testing, Ninth Circuit Court of Appeals Decision, p. 19,839; http://www.reason.com/news/show/117583.html.

She said she wanted to ban the sale: "Teens' dietary aids at issue; Sales to minors of performance-boosting substances would be restricted," *Sacramento Bee*, April 22, 2004.

After spending $22 million: *The People's Machine*, pp. 185-186, 192.

Testosterone was C-Pure: "Papers Detail Trail of Doping," *Los Angeles Times*, June 22, 2004.

Instead, Tygart wrote: "USADA Eases Proof Standard; Move Could Affect BALCO Scandal," *The Washington Post*, June 13,

2004; "Due Process? Not for Track Stars," *The Washington Post*, June 26, 2004.

They were the first cases brought entirely: "World's Fastest Man Faces Lifetime Ban; Lawyers Vow to Fight Agency's 'Lack of Fairness'," *The Mercury News*, June 24, 2004.

"Your failure to commit": "Baseball union chief clever, pathetic in Senate hearing," The Associated Press, March 11, 2004.

The previous month, the House passed: "House votes to ban more supplements," *San Francisco Chronicle*, June 4, 2004.

The Senate bill exempted DHEA: "Steroid Bill Would Exempt Popular Product," *National Journal's Congress Daily*, May 14, 2004.

But the anti-aging market: "Healthy, Wealthy, But Wise?" *Los Angeles Times Magazine*, February 1, 2004.

"I won't recommend it": "DHEA: Ignore the Hype," *HealthNews*, November 19, 1996.

The American Academy of Anti-Aging Medicine: http://www. worldhealth.net/p/4186,5715.html.

Ironically, business was never better: Interview with Arnold.

They sold shirts: http://forum.bodybuilding.com/archive/index. php/t-183453.html.

Eight days earlier, Congress finally passed: "Sen. Biden Measure to Ban Designer Steroids Becomes Law," *US Fed News*, October 22, 2004.

"[Stallone] wants to be that leader": "Pumping Up Supplements; Arnold's Fitness Expo Above Steroid Scandal," *Daily News* (New York), March 8, 2004.

Lewis lived in Colleyville: Adapted from an unpublished *ESPN The Magazine* article written by Craig Offman. Also, author interview with Lori Lewis.

"The woman said she asked her son": "Steroid Use Suspected in Some Area Schools," *The Courier*, October 1, 2004.

The Panthers were so dispirited: "Grapevine's 'D' dominates late," *Fort Worth Star Telegram*, November 6, 2004.

CHAPTER EIGHTEEN

Proving that the lab owners: Interview with Jack "MacGregor"; general background details from special agent Dan Simmons, public information officer, DEA, San Diego.

He formed a group called the American Academy: "The Guru of Growth," *ESPN The Magazine*, November 11, 2006; "The Forever Young Issue; A Drug's Promise (or Not) of Youth," *Los Angeles Times*, July 9, 2006.

His World Congress on Anti-Aging: "Anti-aging industry rolls out its latest gadgets at meeting here," *Chicago Sun-Times*, August 23, 2004.

The FDA, of course, disagreed: "Anti-aging movement fuels interest in HGH," ESPN.com, June 19, 2006.

In response to a Freedom of Information Act request: The FOIA was filed by this writer.

Bruce Kneller sped down a rural road: All details from interview with Kneller.

The law specifically banned: http://www.theorator.com/bills108/hr3866.html.

He reportedly had tried to call: "Baseball stars, Leadership Grilled by House Panel," *The Frontrunner*, March 18, 2005.

The league also waited until the last minute: "McGwire declines to appear before House committee," *St. Louis Post-Dispatch*, March 9, 2005.

McGwire sent word that he "respectfully declined": Ibid.

They refused to take the same oath: "Professional Baseball Players Testify about Steroids," CNN, *Inside Politics*, March 17, 2005.

There was a time, early on: http://insider.espn.go.com/proxy/proxy.dll/insider/magazine/story?id=1940435&action=login&appRedirect=http%3a%2f%2finsider.espn.go.com%2fproxy%2fproxy.dll%2finsider%2fmagazine%2fstory%3fid%3d1940435.

"All that shows me": "Last Laugh," *ESPN The Magazine*, December 20, 2004.

Even if the BALCO men had been convicted: "BALCO prosecutors fumbled the ball," *San Francisco Chronicle*, July 17, 2005.

Anderson would plead guilty: "40 of 42 BALCO charges dropped," *San Francisco Chronicle*, July 16, 2005; "Two sentenced to prison for providing performance-enhancing drugs to professional athletes," *US Fed News*, October 19, 2005.

While two judges would rule: US v. Comprehensive Drug Testing, p. 19,866.

As shoppers began filling: Interview with "McGregor."

"You are cowards": "Steroids in baseball, Players denounce drugs," *The Providence Journal*, March 18, 2004.

They arranged for sales: US v. Denkall, indictment, page 25.

Hooton, a marketing executive: "MLB Gives $1M to 'Roid Charity," *New York Post*, August 19, 2005.

The Mexican steroid trade wasn't going to die: "The Mexican Connection," *Sports Illustrated*, April 24, 2006.

CHAPTER NINETEEN

Now on this wintry morning: Interview with Kneller; all other details from Norfolk (Mass.) District Attorney's Office.

When those initiatives came to a vote: "Voters Reject Schwarzenegger's Bid to Remake State Government," *Los Angeles Times*, November 9, 2005.

After his multimillion dollar publishing deal: "Gov. to Be Paid $8 Million by Fitness Magazines," *Los Angeles Times*, July 14, 2005.

It expanded on a bill: "Governor signs bills aimed at teen behavior," *San Francisco Chronicle*, October 8, 2005.

"That was one of the biggest adrenaline rushes": "Yankee Ends Real Corker of a Mystery," *The New York Times*, April 11, 1999.

The pitcher answered his door: Novitzky affidavit in support of warrant to search home of Jason Grimsley, May 31, 2006, Attachment A.

With friends still inside: Ibid., p. 2.

With that list and the secret memo: "Report: Independent Investigation, Analysis Samples from the 1999 Tour de France," author Emile Vrijman.

In Hamilton's case: "Irreconcilable differences between the results from the Athens sample and the Vuelta sample," brief submitted by Tyler Hamilton before the Court of Arbitration for Sport.

The New York Times **gave the story:** "Cheating or an Early Mingling of the Blood?" *The New York Times*, May 10, 2005.

The conversations that were underway: Interview with Madden.

"It's the sort of thing that motivates people": "Landis Has a Lock on Tour," *Los Angeles Times*, July 23, 2006.

Five months after: Author interview with Howard Jacobs.

Before another bombshell hit: "Track and Field World Is Reeling Over Gatlin," *The New York Times*, July 31, 2006.

The A-sample Jones provided: Author interview with Allen K. Murray, a California biochemist hired by Jones to watch the retest.

After Ma was removed: "Sports administrators push Liaoning hard over doping scandal," *Xinhua General News Service*, August 25, 2006.

Late in the morning: "China probes into 'collective doping' by sports school," *Xinhua General News Service*, August 23, 2006. Author interview with Zhao Jian, Chinese Anti-Doping Agency.

And 141 bottles of steroids: "Doped Chinese sports student as young as 15, official," *Xinhua General News Service*, August 24, 2006.

"We support the decisions": "Sports administrators push Liaoning hard over doping scandal," *Xinhua General News Service*, August 25, 2006.

Of the more than 250 tests given: "Four more Chinese athletes caught doping," *Agence France Presse*, September 7, 2006.

The previous week in Milwaukee: "Bonds breaks Aaron's NL home run record with No. 734," The Associated Press, September 24, 2006.

The other camp: "Legal sideshow, not home run hoopla, follows Bonds," *The New York Times*, February 17, 2007.

A judge ordered him back to jail: "Bonds trainer back behind bars," *San Francisco Chronicle*, August 29, 2006.

"I believe all 30 teams would be interested": "Bonds' agent set for offers," *San Francisco Chronicle*, October 31, 2006.

"There are other labs starting up": "Gear on the Street," *Muscular Development*, February 2007.

CHAPTER TWENTY

Since its release in late December: "Muscle in middle bulks up pic biz," *Daily Variety*, December 29, 2006.

On an international tour: "Sylvester Stallone attends British premier of his new film," The Associated Press, January 16, 2007.

As he stepped off a Qantas flight: "Stallone tried to import HGH, court told," *Bulletin Wire*, March 13, 2007.

When Stallone's luggage was randomly X-rayed: "Sly defends smuggling rap," *The Evening Standard*, April 24, 2007.

"Where do you think": "Rambo feeling rocky—Stallone begs for leniency on steroids charges," *The Daily Telegraph* (Australia), May 16, 2007.

Of course, the authors of the study noted: Garvan Institute of Medical Research press release, June 4, 2007.

The doctor's name was familiar: "Sylvester Stallone fined," The Associated Press, May 22, 2007.

A beautiful obstetrician: http://www.agelesshealth.org/ag-about_dr.htm.

The meeting had been arranged: "2 plead guilty in steroids case," *The Times Union*, April 21, 2007; author interview with Albany District Attorney's Office. Also, author interview with Christopher Baynes, assistant district attorney (Albany, New York).

According to a report: "World Traffic in Doping Substances," Alessandro Donati, Report to World Anti-Doping Agency, February 2007, p. 90.

His main job was, of all things: Author interview with the importer, whose name is withheld at his request.

A medical correspondent: http://www.agelesshealth.org/ag-about_dr.htm.

One invoice showed: According to a source who saw the records.

Another reportedly showed: "RX for Trouble: Inside the Steroid Ring," *Sports Illustrated*, March 12, 2007; Matthews proclaims that he's never taken HGH," ESPN.com, March 15, 2007.

Though dropped from the team's roster: "Steelers drop longtime MD," *Pittsburgh Post-Gazette*, June 15, 2007.

"Clearly, steroid use is something": "Bodybuilding connection again singes governor," *San Francisco Chronicle*, March 6, 2007.

In the end, scores of patients: "Serono Settlement Should Highlight Need for Compliance," *FDA Advertising and Promotion Manual*, December 2005, Vol. 13, No. 10.

"The numbers in the weight room": "SCIL looking into new alignment for next year," *Daily Record*, September 12, 2006.

The Chatham coaches: Author interview with Sal Marinello, Chatham High School coach.

Morris County police arrested 54 people: "Suspect's dad: Steroid, drug charges exaggerated," *Daily Record*, March 13, 2007.

Both men were charged: "Police nab 16 in suburban steroid ring," *The Star Ledger*, March 13, 2007; news release from the Morris County Prosecutor's Office, March 12, 2007.

"We're finding a lot of kids": "Steroid use among teens troubles Web investigators," *Palm Beach Post*, March 25, 2007.

Meanwhile, a Florida legislator: "High school steroid testing earns full committee backing," *Palm Beach Post*, March 7, 2007.

"Totally innocent of doping": Author interview with Michael Henson, Floyd Fairness Fund.

The problem is at the root: "Riding hard at restoring his integrity," *The Mercury News*, February 18, 2007.

"You've got a code of ethics": "Landis case succeeds in exposing faults," *Los Angeles Times*, May 31, 2007.

"That man [Landis] is innocent": "Floyd Fans Treated Unfairly," ESPN.com, May 19, 2007.

"If I did, it would destroy a lot of my friends": USADA v. Floyd Landis, arbitration hearing transcript, pp. 605-607.

He confided that he had been sexually abused: Ibid., p. 613.

"I figured this was an intimidation": Ibid., pp. 615-616.

But LeMond's attorney cut him off: Ibid., pp. 623-624.

"I don't think he did it": "Armstrong: Landis is innocent of doping," The Associated Press, July 5, 2007.

"Well, then he's got to be dirty, too": "Armstrong won't attend Tour, but 'I still love what it represents,'" The Associated Press, July 6, 2007.

In May, Denmark's Bjarne Riis: "1996 Tour de France Champ Admits Doping," The Associated Press, May 26, 2007.

Italian authorities announced that Ivan Basso: "Basso confesses to role in doping scandal," *The Daily Telegraph* (London), May 8, 2007.

And German investigators continued their probe: "IOC: Ulrich would lose 2000 Olympic gold if doping allegations proved," The Associated Press, June 12, 2007.

"What we should have done": "Giambi says Bonds getting bad rap," *USA Today*, May 18, 2007.

Greg Anderson was sitting mute in a jail cell: "Appeals court orders Bonds' trainer to jail," *Los Angeles Times*, November 17, 2006.

As with another infamous affidavit: Jeff Novitzky affidavit in support of a warrant to search Kirk Radomski's home, December 13, 2005, p. 15.

Over the past 20 years: Statistic from *Wrestling Babylon: Piledriving Tales of Drugs, Sex, Death, and Scandal,* by Irvin Muchnick.

At one point, his wife, Nancy: "Chris Benoit's Final Days," *People*, July 16, 2007.

INDEX

A

G

H

About the Author

Shaun Assael is an award-winning investigative writer with *ESPN The Magazine.* He is the author of *Wide Open,* a chronicle of the 1996 NASCAR season, and co-author (with Mike Mooneyham) of an unauthorized biography of the WWE's Vince McMahon, *Sex, Lies, and Headlocks,* which was a *New York Times* bestseller.